Synthesis Lectures on Biomedical Engineering

This series consists of concise books on advanced and state-of-the-art topics that span the field of biomedical engineering. Each Lecture covers the fundamental principles in a unified manner, develops underlying concepts needed for sequential material, and progresses to more advanced topics and design. The authors selected to write the Lectures are leading experts on the subject who have extensive background in theory, application, and design. The series is designed to meet the demands of the 21st century technology and the rapid advancements in the all-encompassing field of biomedical engineering.

Sudip Mukherjee · Boram Kim · Andrea Hernandez

Immunomodulatory Biomaterials for Cell Therapy and Tissue Engineering

Recent Advancements

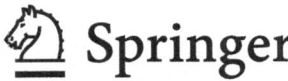

Sudip Mukherjee
School of Biomedical Engineering
Indian Institute of Technology (BHU)
Varanasi, India

Boram Kim
Department of Bioengineering
Rice University
Houston, TX, USA

Andrea Hernandez
The University of Texas MD Anderson Cancer Center
Houston, TX, USA

ISSN 1930-0328   ISSN 1930-0336 (electronic)
Synthesis Lectures on Biomedical Engineering
ISBN 978-3-031-50846-2   ISBN 978-3-031-50844-8 (eBook)
https://doi.org/10.1007/978-3-031-50844-8

© The Editor(s) (if applicable) and The Author(s), under exclusive license to Springer Nature Switzerland AG 2024

This work is subject to copyright. All rights are solely and exclusively licensed by the Publisher, whether the whole or part of the material is concerned, specifically the rights of translation, reprinting, reuse of illustrations, recitation, broadcasting, reproduction on microfilms or in any other physical way, and transmission or information storage and retrieval, electronic adaptation, computer software, or by similar or dissimilar methodology now known or hereafter developed.
The use of general descriptive names, registered names, trademarks, service marks, etc. in this publication does not imply, even in the absence of a specific statement, that such names are exempt from the relevant protective laws and regulations and therefore free for general use.
The publisher, the authors, and the editors are safe to assume that the advice and information in this book are believed to be true and accurate at the date of publication. Neither the publisher nor the authors or the editors give a warranty, expressed or implied, with respect to the material contained herein or for any errors or omissions that may have been made. The publisher remains neutral with regard to jurisdictional claims in published maps and institutional affiliations.

This Springer imprint is published by the registered company Springer Nature Switzerland AG
The registered company address is: Gewerbestrasse 11, 6330 Cham, Switzerland

Paper in this product is recyclable.

Contents

1 **Introduction: Immune Response to the Implanted Biomaterial** 1
  Boram Kim and Sudip Mukherjee
  1.1 Introduction 1
  1.2 Immune Response to the Implanted Biomaterial 2
  1.3 Immunomodulation Using Biological Molecules or Cells 4
  References 6

2 **Immunomodulation Strategies Using Biomaterial Chemistry and Physical Properties** 9
  Sudip Mukherjee
  2.1 Introduction 9
  2.2 Immunomodulation by Biomaterial Chemistry 10
      2.2.1 Non-Biofouling Methodologies 11
      2.2.2 Bioinspired Extracellular Matrix (ECM) Elements 15
      2.2.3 Zwitterionic Biomaterials for Immunomodulation 15
  2.3 Impact of Biomaterial's Physical Properties on Immunomodulation 16
      2.3.1 Effect of Surface Topography on Immunomodulation 16
      2.3.2 Impact of the Implant Geometry on Immunomodulation 18
      2.3.3 Impact of the Implant Mechanical Properties on Immunomodulation 20
  References 21

3 **Use of Immunomodulatory Biomaterials in Diabetes Therapy** 25
  Boram Kim and Sudip Mukherjee
  3.1 Introduction 25
  3.2 Conventional Therapies in Diabetes and Limitations 26
  3.3 Cell Therapies for Diabetes and Their Challenges 27
  3.4 Graft Failure 29
  3.5 Development of Immunomodulatory Biomaterials for Diabetes Therapy 29
  References 36

4	**Cell-Based Therapies in Cancer**	39
	Andrea Hernandez and Sudip Mukherjee	
	4.1 Introduction	39
	4.2 Fundamentals of Cancer Immunology and Immunotherapy	40
	4.3 Ovarian Cancers and Aplated Ovaries	43
	4.4 Colorectal Cancer	50
	4.5 Melanoma	50
	4.6 Other Cancers	54
	4.7 Conclusions	56
	References	58
5	**Cell-Based Therapies in Myocardial Infarction and Tissue Regeneration**	61
	Andrea Hernandez and Sudip Mukherjee	
	5.1 Introduction	61
	5.2 Cell-Based Therapies in Myocardial Infarction	63
	5.3 Tissue Regeneration	69
	5.4 Conclusions	76
	References	76
6	**Recent Clinical Trials on Immunomodulatory Biomaterials Applications**	79
	Sudip Mukherjee	
	6.1 Clinical Trials	79
	6.2 Conclusion and Future Perspectives	84
	References	85

Introduction: Immune Response to the Implanted Biomaterial

Boram Kim and Sudip Mukherjee

1.1 Introduction

Cell therapy and tissue engineering have emerged as a revolutionary approach in medicine, with the potential to restore malfunctioning tissues and treat a wide range of diseases in a way that traditional drugs cannot achieve [2]. These therapies involve various sources of cells and show promise in treating cancer [3], diabetes [4], and autoimmune disorders [5, 6]. However, the immune response of the recipient's body poses a significant challenge to the widespread adoption and success of cell-based therapies. To address this challenge, biomaterials have been used as invaluable tools in healthcare applications, particularly in drug delivery for immune system regulation and the isolation of transplanted cells. The use of biomaterials in drug delivery, cell therapy, and tissue engineering offers several advantages, including targeted delivery of therapeutics, reduced drug toxicity, minimized side effects, reduced reliance on immunosuppressive agents, and the ability to customize drug and cell-based therapies [2, 7–9]. Despite these advancements, current strategies face limitations, such as a lack of sustained therapeutic effects and immune reactions to biomaterials known as foreign body responses (FBRs). These immune responses can lead to delayed healing, inflammation, rejection of medical implants, and tissue damage [10]. In the case of biomaterials containing live cells, inflammation can hinder the transfer of tissue mass. Overcoming these challenges requires innovative strategies to predict

B. Kim
Department of Bioengineering, Rice University Houston, TX, USA

S. Mukherjee (✉)
School of Biomedical Engineering, Indian Institute of Technology (BHU), Varanasi 221005, UP, India
e-mail: sudip.bme@iitbhu.ac.in

the fate of biomaterials after implantation, modulate immune responses, and minimize side effects caused by the host immune system and FBRs. Immunomodulatory biomaterials are emerging as a new approach to revolutionize cell and organ transplantation. Design strategies for biomaterials are now used to induce a tolerogenic response instead of relying on immunosuppression, resulting in long-lasting and targeted immune regulation [1, 11]. Moreover, biomaterials can be customized to engage specific immune cell subsets by manipulating their surface and chemical properties, promoting a favorable immune response [7, 12]. Temporal control over the deployment of specific cells and immune suppression during crucial events can also be achieved using immunomodulatory biomaterials. This book aims to provide a comprehensive overview of recent advancements in immunomodulatory biomaterials for various biomedical applications. We explore the characteristics of biomaterials that play a crucial role in triggering specific immune responses. Furthermore, we emphasize the use of immunomodulatory biomaterials in treating different diseases such as diabetes, cancer, and tissue regeneration.

1.2 Immune Response to the Implanted Biomaterial

When a biomaterial is implanted into the body, the immune system recognizes it as a foreign object and initiates a series of immune responses. These foreign body response (FBRs) to biomaterials involves a complex series of immune reactions and tissue remodeling processes that can lead to the formation of fibrous capsules, granulomas, and fibrosis, ultimately affecting the success of implanted biomaterials and therapies. The temporal sequence of host immune responses to implanted biomaterials can be broadly categorized into four phases: protein adsorption, acute inflammation, chronic inflammation, and tissue remodeling (Fig. 1.1a). First, upon implantation, proteins from the surrounding biological fluids and blood immediately start to adsorb onto the surface of the biomaterial. Within minutes, proteins from the blood and platelets form a clot around the biomaterial, which contains various cytokines, growth factors, and attractants that recruit immune cells to the site [13]. Immune cells, such as neutrophils and mast cells, are recruited to the implant site. Neutrophils are the first responders and release inflammatory mediators, such as cytokines and chemokines, to amplify the inflammatory response [14–16]. This phase typically resolves within a week, depending on the extent of the injury. Mast cell degranulation and fibrinogen adsorption play a role in the acute inflammatory response to the biomaterial [17, 18]. As the transition from acute to chronic inflammation occurs, monocytes migrate to the site and transform into macrophages. Monocytes differentiate into macrophages (M1), which release pro-inflammatory factors to eliminate the foreign material [19, 20]. Macrophages adhere to the biomaterial surface and attempt to degrade it through phagocytosis. However, some biomaterials may resist degradation, leading to the persistence of macrophages at the implant site. The activated macrophages release additional inflammatory mediators, which can attract more immune cells and further amplify the inflammatory response [13]. Lymphocytes, particularly T cells, become more prominent in the chronic inflammation phase. T cells play a role in adaptive immunity and can recognize specific antigens presented by the biomaterial or antigen-presenting cells [21]. In ideal situations, an initial chronic inflammatory response dominated by M1 macrophages is followed by a transition to a pro-healing environment with an abundance of M2 macrophages [22]. The M2 macrophages release anti-inflammatory factors that help resolve inflammation and promote tissue regeneration [21]. However, if the transition from M1 macrophages to M2 macrophages, which are involved in tissue repair and resolution of inflammation, is impaired, the chronic presence of M1 macrophages and persistent inflammation can lead to an exaggerated immune response [7]. This can result in the formation of a fibrous capsule around the biomaterial, fusion of macrophages to form foreign body giant cells (FBGCs), and the recruitment of other cells, such as myofibroblasts [7]. The myofibroblasts produce excessive amounts of pro-fibrogenic and extracellular matrix proteins, including collagen, leading to the formation of granulomas and fibrosis [23]. The fibrotic tissue restricts the diffusion of soluble factors, compromising the delivery of nutrients and oxygen to the surrounding cells, including the transplanted cells [23]. This limited diffusion and impaired tissue environment can ultimately result in the death of transplanted cells and failure of the therapy [23, 24] (Fig. 1.1b).

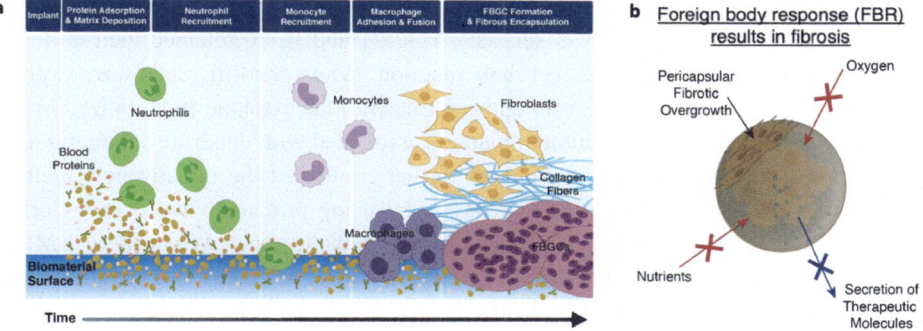

Fig. 1.1 a Temporal sequence of host immune responses to foreign materials. First, circulating proteins adhere to the biomaterial surface, triggering immune recognition by recruited neutrophils and monocytes. Adhered macrophages begin to fuse and form foreign body giant cells (FBGCs) (Adapted from Kim, et al. [1]). b Foreign body response (FBR) results in fibrosis capsule formation, which leads to graft failure

1.3 Immunomodulation Using Biological Molecules or Cells

As mentioned earlier, when biomaterials are implanted, they trigger host immune responses known as FBRs, which affects the integration and performance of the implant [25]. This response involves various inflammatory reactions and the recruitment of immune cells to the implant site [9, 26]. The properties of the biomaterials themselves also play a role in influencing the behavior of macrophages, which in turn affect tissue healing [9, 25, 27]. Consequently, researchers have developed immunomodulatory materials that can control the immune response at the implantation site. Delivering biological molecules or cells within biomaterials can alter local immune responses to the implant site. One approach involves incorporating anti-inflammatory drugs or cytokines into the biomaterial substrates to regulate the interaction between immune cells and the surrounding tissues. Cytokines and growth factors have the ability to influence the behavior of immune cells, making them promising candidates for sustained release from bioactive coatings [7]. These molecules can be delivered locally by immobilizing them within the biomaterial, such as hydrogels, or by using nucleic-acid-based methods that allow for prolonged synthesis and release of cytokines by cells implanted in situ [7]. For example, incorporating TGF-β or IL-10 into hydrogels has been effective in suppressing the maturation of dendritic cells [25, 28]. Hume et al. [28] utilized a cytokine-based strategy to modify poly(ethylene glycol) (PEG) hydrogels by immobilizing immunosuppressive cytokines (TGF-β1 and IL-10) on the hydrogel surfaces. These two cytokines are commonly used in vitro to influence the behavior of dendritic cells. The researchers demonstrated that even when attached to the hydrogel surfaces, TGF-β1 and IL-10 retained their ability to interact with dendritic cells and affect their function. When dendritic cells were exposed to lipopolysaccharide or cytokines while interacting with the cytokine-immobilized hydrogels, there was a noticeable reduction in markers associated with dendritic cell maturation, such as IL-12 and MHCII. The researchers further confirmed the effectiveness of these hydrogels in modulating dendritic cell behavior by using primary bone marrow-derived dendritic cells (BMDCs) obtained from non-obese diabetic mice. When these BMDCs interacted with the immunosuppressive hydrogels, there was a decrease in activation markers and a significant decrease in their ability to activate T cells. This approach shows promise for the development of biomaterials that can regulate immune responses and foster tolerance, particularly in the field of cell-based therapeutics. Sequential controlled delivery of IFN-γ and IL-4 from scaffolds or double hydrogel layers has been shown to promote the transition of macrophages from the M1 pro-inflammatory phenotype to the M2 pro-healing phenotype [25, 29, 30].

Additionally, the delivery of pharmacological anti-inflammatory agents like heparin, dexamethasone, and superoxide dismutase from reservoirs and coatings has demonstrated the ability to reduce inflammation and fibrous encapsulation [21, 31, 32]. Also, a strategy involving the binding of immunomodulatory agents to the surrounding biomaterial can be employed instead of relying on drug release into the surrounding environment [8]. This approach enables targeted and localized immunomodulation while minimizing negative effects on the encapsulated cells and preventing the agents from diffusing away from the implantation site. For example, by linking streptavidin-Fas ligand (FasL) to short PEG chains attached to pancreatic islets, the apoptosis mechanism dependent on Fas-FasL can be utilized [33]. Coating the islets with FasL, along with the systemic administration of rapamycin for a two-week period, effectively prevents rejection of the allograft and stimulates increased migration of regulatory T cells into the graft, surpassing the response seen with unmodified islets. Additionally, PEG microbeads coated with cell-free FasL can be co-transplanted with uncoated islets, resulting in enhanced protection of the allograft when combined with two weeks of systemic rapamycin delivery [34, 35]. These studies demonstrated the successful promotion of immunomodulation by the FasL-engineered biomaterials, leading to the acceptance of allogeneic islet grafts in animal models.

Another strategy involves cell therapy, where immune cells are included to produce specific molecules or induce biological events, or their recruitment is stimulated [7]. The immunoregulatory properties of mesenchymal stem cells (MSCs) have been extensively studied. Encapsulated MSCs have been shown to attenuate the fibrotic response compared to acellular hydrogels by downregulating pro-inflammatory macrophages [36]. Based on the immunomodulatory properties of MSCs and their potential in tissue engineering, researchers proposed that encapsulated MSCs within PEG hydrogels could alleviate the for FBR [36]. Authors observed that murine MSCs encapsulated within PEG hydrogels reduced the activation of macrophages in vitro. This was evident from the decreased expression of genes and secretion of pro-inflammatory cytokines, specifically tumor necrosis factor-α. To evaluate the effect of MSCs on the fibrotic response of the FBR in vivo, they implanted hydrogels loaded with MSCs, MSCs undergoing osteogenic differentiation, or no cells into C57BL/6 mice for a duration of 28 days. The presence of encapsulated MSCs resulted in a decrease in the thickness of the fibrous capsule compared to acellular hydrogels. However, this effect diminished when the MSCs underwent osteogenic differentiation. Through continuous communication between MSCs and inflammatory cells, it is feasible to regulate macrophage activation and mitigate the FBR to implanted materials, consequently enhancing long-term biomaterials funtions [36]. These strategies aim to modulate the inflammatory response and promote a favorable environment for tissue healing and integration of the biomaterials. By manipulating the release of bioactive molecules or incorporating specific cell types, it is possible to regulate the immune response and enhance the performance of implanted biomaterials.

References

1. Kim, B. *et al.* Current Advances in Immunomodulatory Biomaterials for Cell Therapy and Tissue Engineering. *Advanced Therapeutics* **n/a**, 2300002, https://doi.org/10.1002/adtp.202300002.
2. Chua, C. Y. X. *et al.* Emerging immunomodulatory strategies for cell therapeutics. *Trends in Biotechnology* **41**, 358-373, https://doi.org/10.1016/j.tibtech.2022.11.008 (2023).
3. Sterner, R. C. & Sterner, R. M. CAR-T cell therapy: current limitations and potential strategies. *Blood Cancer Journal* **11**, 69, https://doi.org/10.1038/s41408-021-00459-7 (2021).
4. Pires, I. G. S., Silva e Souza, J. A., de Melo Bisneto, A. V., Passos, X. S. & Carneiro, C. C. Clinical efficacy of stem-cell therapy on diabetes mellitus: A systematic review and meta-analysis. *Transplant Immunology* **75**, 101740, https://doi.org/10.1016/j.trim.2022.101740 (2022).
5. Aghajanian, H., Rurik, J. G. & Epstein, J. A. CAR-based therapies: opportunities for immuno-medicine beyond cancer. *Nature Metabolism* **4**, 163-169, https://doi.org/10.1038/s42255-022-00537-5 (2022).
6. Ghobadinezhad, F. *et al.* The emerging role of regulatory cell-based therapy in autoimmune disease. *Front Immunol* **13**, 1075813, https://doi.org/10.3389/fimmu.2022.1075813 (2022).
7. Vishwakarma, A. *et al.* Engineering Immunomodulatory Biomaterials To Tune the Inflammatory Response. *Trends in Biotechnology* **34**, 470-482, https://doi.org/10.1016/j.tibtech.2016.03.009 (2016).
8. Stabler, C. L., Li, Y., Stewart, J. M. & Keselowsky, B. G. Engineering immunomodulatory biomaterials for type 1 diabetes. *Nature Reviews Materials* **4**, 429-450, https://doi.org/10.1038/s41578-019-0112-5 (2019).
9. Lee, J., Byun, H., Madhurakkat Perikamana, S. K., Lee, S. & Shin, H. Current Advances in Immunomodulatory Biomaterials for Bone Regeneration. *Adv Healthc Mater* **8**, 1801106, https://doi.org/10.1002/adhm.201801106 (2019).
10. Veiseh, O. & Vegas, A. J. Domesticating the foreign body response: Recent advances and applications. *Advanced Drug Delivery Reviews* **144**, 148-161, https://doi.org/10.1016/j.addr.2019.08.010 (2019).
11. Hotaling, N. A., Tang, L., Irvine, D. J. & Babensee, J. E. Biomaterial Strategies for Immunomodulation. *Annu Rev Biomed Eng* **17**, 317-349, https://doi.org/10.1146/annurev-bioeng-071813-104814 (2015).
12. Orive, G. *et al.* Engineering a Clinically Translatable Bioartificial Pancreas to Treat Type I Diabetes. *Trends in Biotechnology* **36**, 445-456, https://doi.org/10.1016/j.tibtech.2018.01.007 (2018).
13. Mariani, E., Lisignoli, G., Borzì, R. M. & Pulsatelli, L. Biomaterials: Foreign Bodies or Tuners for the Immune Response? *Int J Mol Sci* **20**, https://doi.org/10.3390/ijms20030636 (2019).
14. Sheikh, Z., Brooks, P. J., Barzilay, O., Fine, N. & Glogauer, M. Macrophages, Foreign Body Giant Cells and Their Response to Implantable Biomaterials. *Materials (Basel)* **8**, 5671-5701, https://doi.org/10.3390/ma8095269 (2015).
15. Lock, A., Cornish, J. & Musson, D. S. The Role of In Vitro Immune Response Assessment for Biomaterials. *J Funct Biomater* **10**, 31, https://doi.org/10.3390/jfb10030031 (2019).
16. Kolaczkowska, E. & Kubes, P. Neutrophil recruitment and function in health and inflammation. *Nature Reviews Immunology* **13**, 159-175, https://doi.org/10.1038/nri3399 (2013).
17. Anderson, J. M., Rodriguez, A. & Chang, D. T. Foreign body reaction to biomaterials. *Seminars in Immunology* **20**, 86-100, https://doi.org/10.1016/j.smim.2007.11.004 (2008).

18. Luster, A. D., Alon, R. & von Andrian, U. H. Immune cell migration in inflammation: present and future therapeutic targets. *Nature Immunology* **6**, 1182-1190, https://doi.org/10.1038/ni1275 (2005).
19. Gordon, S. & Taylor, P. R. Monocyte and macrophage heterogeneity. *Nature Reviews Immunology* **5**, 953-964, https://doi.org/10.1038/nri1733 (2005).
20. Soehnlein, O. & Lindbom, L. Phagocyte partnership during the onset and resolution of inflammation. *Nature Reviews Immunology* **10**, 427-439, https://doi.org/10.1038/nri2779 (2010).
21. Udipi, K. *et al.* Modification of inflammatory response to implanted biomedical materials in vivo by surface bound superoxide dismutase mimics. *Journal of Biomedical Materials Research* **51**, 549-560, https://doi.org/10.1002/1097-4636(20000915)51:4<549::AID-JBM2>3.0.CO;2-Z (2000).
22. Davies, L. C., Jenkins, S. J., Allen, J. E. & Taylor, P. R. Tissue-resident macrophages. *Nature Immunology* **14**, 986-995, https://doi.org/10.1038/ni.2705 (2013).
23. Bashor, C. J., Hilton, I. B., Bandukwala, H., Smith, D. M. & Veiseh, O. Engineering the next generation of cell-based therapeutics. *Nature Reviews Drug Discovery* **21**, 655-675, https://doi.org/10.1038/s41573-022-00476-6 (2022).
24. Chandorkar, Y., K, R. & Basu, B. The Foreign Body Response Demystified. *ACS Biomaterials Science & Engineering* **5**, 19–44, https://doi.org/10.1021/acsbiomaterials.8b00252 (2019).
25. Mariani, E., Lisignoli, G., Borzi, R. M. & Pulsatelli, L. Biomaterials: Foreign Bodies or Tuners for the Immune Response? *Int J Mol Sci* **20**, https://doi.org/10.3390/ijms20030636 (2019).
26. Cravedi, P. *et al.* Regenerative immunology: the immunological reaction to biomaterials. *Transplant International* **30**, 1199-1208, https://doi.org/10.1111/tri.13068 (2017).
27. Taraballi, F. *et al.* Biomimetic Tissue Engineering: Tuning the Immune and Inflammatory Response to Implantable Biomaterials. *Adv Healthc Mater* **7**, 1800490, https://doi.org/10.1002/adhm.201800490 (2018).
28. Hume, P. S., He, J., Haskins, K. & Anseth, K. S. Strategies to reduce dendritic cell activation through functional biomaterial design. *Biomaterials* **33**, 3615-3625, https://doi.org/10.1016/j.biomaterials.2012.02.009 (2012).
29. Chen, J. *et al.* Macrophage phenotype switch by sequential action of immunomodulatory cytokines from hydrogel layers on titania nanotubes. *Colloids and Surfaces B: Biointerfaces* **163**, 336-345, https://doi.org/10.1016/j.colsurfb.2018.01.007 (2018).
30. Spiller, K. L. *et al.* Sequential delivery of immunomodulatory cytokines to facilitate the M1-to-M2 transition of macrophages and enhance vascularization of bone scaffolds. *Biomaterials* **37**, 194-207, https://doi.org/10.1016/j.biomaterials.2014.10.017 (2015).
31. Peng, Y., Tellier, L. E. & Temenoff, J. S. Heparin-based hydrogels with tunable sulfation & degradation for anti-inflammatory small molecule delivery. *Biomater Sci* **4**, 1371-1380, https://doi.org/10.1039/c6bm00455e (2016).
32. Zhong, Y. & Bellamkonda, R. V. Dexamethasone-coated neural probes elicit attenuated inflammatory response and neuronal loss compared to uncoated neural probes. *Brain Research* **1148**, 15-27, https://doi.org/10.1016/j.brainres.2007.02.024 (2007).
33. Yolcu, E. S. *et al.* Pancreatic Islets Engineered with SA-FasL Protein Establish Robust Localized Tolerance by Inducing Regulatory T Cells in Mice. *The Journal of Immunology* **187**, 5901-5909, https://doi.org/10.4049/jimmunol.1003266 (2011).

34. Lei, J. *et al*. FasL microgels induce immune acceptance of islet allografts in nonhuman primates. *Science Advances* **8**, eabm9881, https://doi.org/10.1126/sciadv.abm9881 (2022).
35. Headen, D. M. *et al*. Local immunomodulation with Fas ligand-engineered biomaterials achieves allogeneic islet graft acceptance. *Nature Materials* **17**, 732-739, https://doi.org/10.1038/s41563-018-0099-0 (2018).
36. Swartzlander, M. D. *et al*. Immunomodulation by mesenchymal stem cells combats the foreign body response to cell-laden synthetic hydrogels. *Biomaterials* **41**, 79-88, https://doi.org/10.1016/j.biomaterials.2014.11.020 (2015).

Immunomodulation Strategies Using Biomaterial Chemistry and Physical Properties

Sudip Mukherjee

2.1 Introduction

Host immune response can impact biomaterials adversely causing foreign body response (FBR) manipulating the result of the host-integration of the implanted materials. Further, this also significantly affects the overall biological performance and durability of the implant [1]. An implanted biomaterial can elicit no response to the immune system making it biocompatible. On the other hand, the implanted materials may trigger a pro-inflammatory or anti-inflammatory reaction to the host immune system, making them vulnerable for rejection and failure. Interestingly, these inflammatory cascades of different biomolecular signals recruit various immune cells near to the location of the implanted materials [2, 3]. These cells comprise of cytotoxic T cells, B cells, macrophages and other immune cells potentially recognize the threat and process it accordingly. Moreover, physicochemical characteristics of the implanted biomaterials have an important role in the plasticity of macrophages, influencing the tissue healing development [4]. Several instances of biomaterial degradation have led to change of their surface activating the immune system [1]. Hence, researchers and scientists are constantly working on the development of immunomodulatory materials that can tune the immune responses towards them resulting in a better acceptance at the at implantation sites [4]. In this book chapter we will thoroughly cover two focal strategies tuning the inflammatory response of the implanted biomaterials including Sect. 2.2 varying chemical properties of the implanted biomaterials, and Sect. 2.3 alteration of physical characteristics of the

S. Mukherjee (✉)
School of Biomedical Engineering, Indian Institute of Technology (BHU), Varanasi 221005, UP, India
e-mail: sudip.bme@iitbhu.ac.in

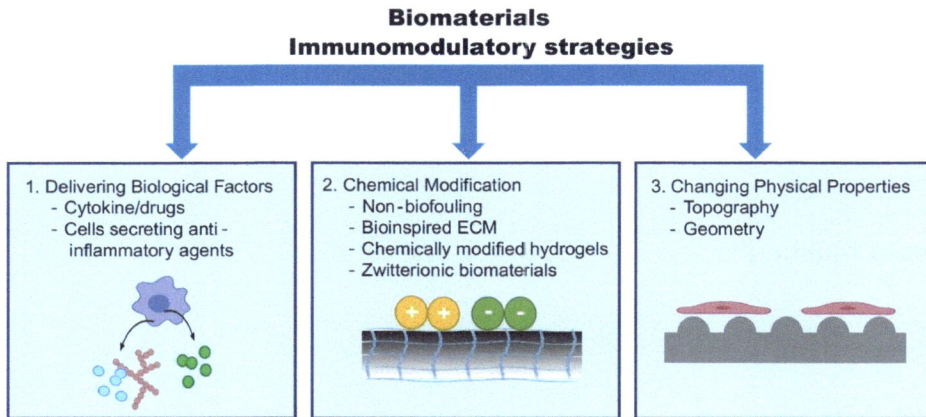

Fig. 2.1 Biomaterial engineering for modulating immune responses. Figure 2.1 is reproduced after permission from @Wiley [5]

implanted biomaterials. Further following subtopics will be consequently covered in detail under the main two above-mentioned sections: Sect. 2.2.1. use of non-biofouling strategies; Sect. 2.2.2 use of bioinspired Extracellular Matrix (ECM) components; Sect. 2.2.3 use of chemically modified hydrogels for immune-isolation of bioactive cells; Sect. 2.2.4 use of zwitterionic biomaterials for immunomodulation; Sect. 2.3.1 role of surface topography in immunomodulation (Texture); Sect. 2.3.2 role of implant/biomaterials geometry in immunomodulation (size and shape) and Sect. 2.3.3 impact of the implant mechanical properties on immunomodulation (Fig. 2.1) [5].

2.2 Immunomodulation by Biomaterial Chemistry

Surface chemistry of biomaterials are an important factor that can be modulated to manipulate the immune reactions to the implanted biomaterials. Surface chemistry can be easily altered with various technologies including, non-biofouling technologies, bioinspired ECM deposition, chemical modification of hydrogels for immune isolation of bioactive cells and zwitterionic based polymeric biomaterials development. Alteration of chemical nature to the implanted biomaterials can change the extent and type of protein absorptions and consequent immunological reactions towards the implant. In this following section we will discuss various strategies that can be utilized to alleviate FBR to the implanted biomaterials and minimize fibrosis.

2.2.1 Non-Biofouling Methodologies

Considerable developments were made for minimization of FBR and reduction of fibrosis to the implanted biomaterials by coating them with immune isolating coating including small molecules, hydrophilic polymeric thin film, etc. [6]. Modification of implanted biomaterials with non-biofouling hydrophilic thin polymeric layers and films has shown tremendous efficacy to inhibit protein attachment and reduction of fibrotic responses, resulting in a higher durability of the implants. Hydrogels with semi-porous nature were utilized to coat to various implanted devices mitigating long-term fibrosis and increasing the durability of the implants due to high water content, accessible solute transmission, and facile surface alteration strategies using suitable chemical moieties [6]. Recent advancement of poly (N-isopropyl acrylamide) (pNIPAm) films fabricated with PEG: to poly (ethylene glycol) were reported to inhibit the attachment of immune sensing macrophages reducing long-term fibrosis. Further it prevents the attachment of leukocyte reducing the secretion of pro-inflammatory cytokines demonstrated by thorough in vivo experiments [6, 7]. Recent developments of cell based therapies have attracted immense attention due to several advantages over chemical drug therapies including long-term efficacy, less side effects, better performance, personalized therapeutic strategies etc. However, the implanted grafts or cellularized constructs require prolonged protection from FBR, which will ensure no significant damage to the cell survival resulting in long-term therapeutic efficacy. Moreover, the hydrogel or biomaterials need to be semi-permeable allowing easy exchange of nutrients, solutes, oxygen, cytokines, oxygen but simultaneously able to prohibit attack from immune cells. Recent studies by Lin and colleagues, demonstrated the use of RGD conjugated PEG followed my attachment of various pro-inflammatory cytokines including TNF-α and MCP-1, influencing enhanced cell survivability compared to unconjugated polymers [8]. This innovative strategy is useful for long-term cell therapy.

Alginate is a naturally derived polymer that can be largely used to prepare biocompatible hydrogel systems for the delivery of therapeutic agents and cells. However, unmodified alginate-based hydrogels have shown FBR when implanted to rodents and humans. To prevent the immune reaction towards the alginates Vegas and Veiseh et al. have utilized the conjugation of immunoprotective small molecules to the surface of the alginates, preventing FBR and mitigating fibrosis. They have employed a large screening strategy and developed a library of 774 chemically modified hydrogels using a diverse range of combinatorial chemistry approaches including very well-known Click Chemistry [9]. Following early screening for anti-inflammatory properties of the hydrogels implanted in the sub-Q space of the mice by measuring the activity of cathepsin (degranulation marker), top 200 lead hydrogel were identified with lower cathepsin activity compared to control alginate. Consequent screening using these top 200 leads narrowed down to top 10 lead hydrogels that showed lowest inflammation and FBR. Detailed analysis using immunostaining, dark-field and phase-contrast microscopy identified three top lead hydrogels with minimum fibrotic tissue deposition following two weeks of intraperitoneal (IP) implantation in mouse model. Moreover, these lead hydrogels also had the lowest amount of collagen, neutrophils, α-smooth muscle actin and macrophage deposition on the surface indicating the role of these innovative chemistry preventing FBR. Intra-vital imaging indicated a significant decrease in macrophage cell population around the lead hydrogel implants compared to the unmodified hydrogels confirming the mechanism of action for lowering the fibrosis levels. Further studies were carried out in non-human primate (NHP) model by implanting 1.5 mm hydrogel capsules of the three leads intraperitoneally demonstrated similar observation with minimum FBR. Mechanical strength and surface roughness were non-significant when tested for the lead small molecule conjugated hydrogels compared to the unmodified indicating the role of chemical functionalization for the reduction of fibrosis. Three lead chemical structures had triazole (heterocyclic five-membered ring containing three nitrogen and two carbon atoms) motif on the backbone, with two of them containing a hydrophilic pegylated linker and the third one had a hydrophobic aromatic ring. This indicates the role of triazole motifs for potential anti-fibrotic and immunoprotective properties of these chemical modifications. Other studies demonstrated the modulation of PEG chain length for the manipulation of antifouling properties of the implanted biomaterials. The variation of terminal groups with polymer chain length, charge, size can be employed to the PEG layer resulting in the changes to the FBR due to varying degree of electrostatic interactions of proteins [10].

In recently published paper by *Mukherjee* et al. the authors demonstrated the synthesis of a second generation of triazole library synthesized by mimicking the structural pattern of the three top leads discovered by *Vegas and Veiseh* [9, 11]. A total of 211 new chemically modified hydrogel analogues were synthesized by varying the alkynes (51 alkynes) and linkers (three hydrophilic PEG2, PEG3 & PEG4 linkers and two hydrophobic linkers containing aromatic functionality). A novel high-throughput screening strategy using cellular barcoding was employed where each hydrogel capsule was barcoded with a distinct donor human umbilical vein endothelial cell (HUVEC). After that, a mixture of 20 different chemically modified hydrogel capsules of 1.5 mm size and containing distinct individual cells were implanted intraperitoneally in immunocompetent C57BL/6 J mouse for 4 weeks (Fig. 2.2). Following the retrieval, the capsules were imaged using dark-field and bright-field to sort the clean capsules without any fibrosis and further extracted DNA from the encapsulated cells were analyzed to determine the cell and material identity.

Using this innovative study, the authors were able to identify new top 10 leads hydrogel with superior anti-fibrotic properties compared to the previously identified 1st generation leads. Additional studies were performed using microcapsules with 0.2 mm size to identify top 3 leads that can show excellent immunoprotective properties. Functional studies were performed to coat medical grade catheters using the one of the top lead hydrophilic and hydrophobic lead small molecules resulted in the low deposition of fibrotic tissues and collagen following 4 weeks implantation in the sub-Q area of mouse (Fig. 2.3)

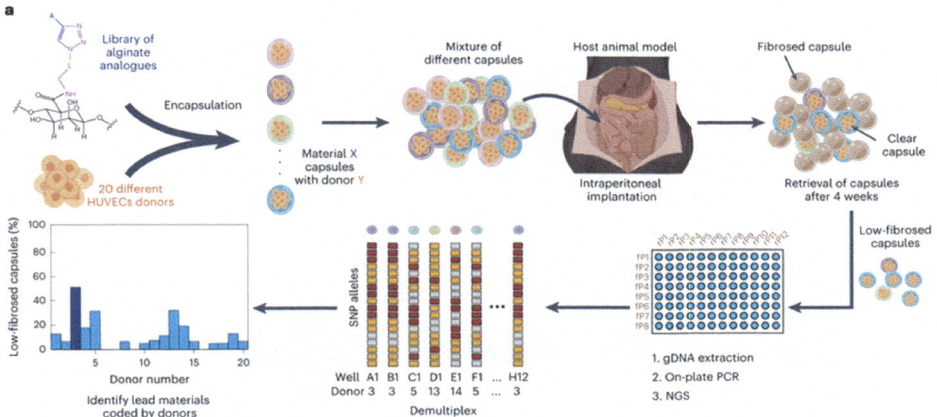

Fig. 2.2 Cell barcoding strategy enables high-throughput materials screening **a**, Overall schematic diagram for the workflow of biomaterials screening: 20 different HUVEC donors were encapsulated with corresponding materials and implanted into mice for evaluating the antifibrotic property and biocompatibility for 4 weeks using NGS assay. The figure is reproduced with permission from Springer Nature [11]

[11]. More studies were performed to deliver xenogeneic human islet cells using lead immunoprotective hydrogels demonstrating restoration of normoglycemia till 3 months when implanted to a type-1 diabetic mouse model. Mechanistic studies revealed that porosity and mechanical strength did not play a significant role in the ability of immunoprotection, further confirming the role of chemical modifications for preventing FBR. In another recent studies from Jason A. Spector and coworkers they utilized innovative small molecule (Met-Z2-Y12 an anti-inflammatory molecule first reported in [9]) coating to silicone breast implants in C57BL/6 mice significantly reducing peri-prosthetic tissue and capsule formation compared to uncoated implants following 21, 90 or 180 days of implantation [12]. The same research group has further reported the combinatory use of Met-Z2-Y12 coating to silicone breast implants along with targeted radiotherapy (20 Gy) caused significant reduction of fibrosis even after 6 months post-implants in a rat model [13].

Rostam et al., identified polymers (with methacrylate and methacrylamide functionalities) using a high-throughput microarray-based screening assay that direct various immune reactions by altering macrophage adhesion resulting the change of polarization from M1 (pro-inflammatory) to M2 (anti-inflammatory) or vice-versa [14]. Further, the coating of the polymers was tested on silicone tubing's towards their in vivo immunological responses in murine model. A machine learning algorithm was utilized to understand the structural relationship between polymer with the cellular responses. Lastly, protein adsorption study was performed that revealed that polymer structures with dense protein adsorbed layer could lead to the pro-inflammatory responses whereas thinner protein

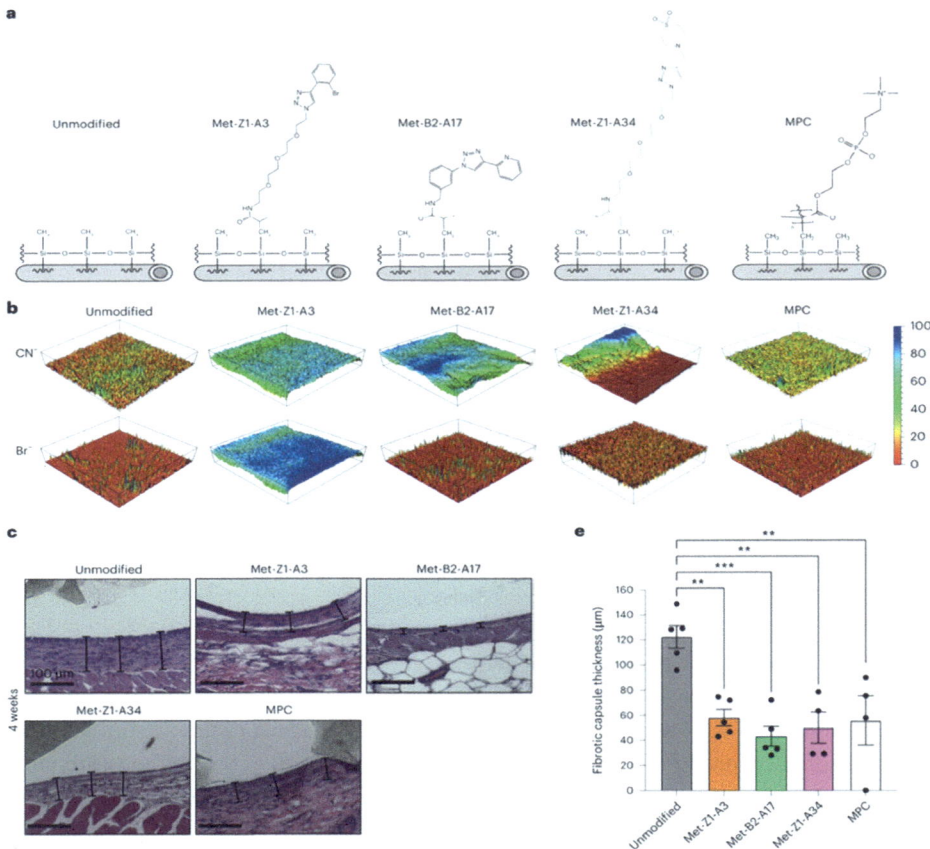

Fig. 2.3 Lead small molecules can be translated for medical applications, including catheter coating **a** Chemical structures of unmodified or coated catheters (coating with either Met-Z1-A3, Met-B2-A17, Met-Z1-A34 or MPC). **b** ToF–SIMS data for unmodified, Met-Z1-A3, Met-B2-A17, Met-Z1-A34 and MPC-modified catheters showing the area with normalized intensity (a.u.) by total ion intensity for the main peaks (CN⁻, Br⁻), indicating successful coating. **c, d,** Representative histology images of the measured fibrotic capsule for unmodified and coated catheters after 4 weeks **c** and 8 weeks **d**. The figure is reproduced with permission from Springer Nature [11]

layer had led to anti-inflammatory response. In another interesting work, A.M. Ghaemmaghami and coworkers screened a diverse library of monosaccharides to show few selective molecules suppressed lipopolysaccharide-stimulated activation of DCs supported by decrease in IL-12, CD40 and indoleamine 2,3-dioxygenase activity but increasing IL-10 amount promoting anti-inflammatory downstream cascade [15].

2.2.2 Bioinspired Extracellular Matrix (ECM) Elements

Extracellular matrix (ECM) incorporation and modification to the implanted biomaterials mimicking the natural microenvironment has shown incredible results inhibiting pro-inflammation and M1-macrophage activation, reducing FBR and triggering wound repair [16]. Kajahn and coworkers reported that enormously sulfated hyaluronan (HA) modified biomaterials shows inhibition of M1-macrophage activation stimulated by the secretion of MCP-1, IFN-γ and IL-6, resulting in the facilitated wound repair close to the implants [17]. Much recent research are focused to develop ECM mimicking surfaces preventing immune activation, macrophage activation, reduction of pro-inflammatory cascades and capsule formation to the implants thus improving the biocompatibility, host acceptance and long-term durability [18]. Further various biological signaling molecules present in both the intrinsic ECM and ECM-mimicking biomaterials inspire such developments. Additional research needs to be performed to examine the role of various structural and soluble ingredients present in the ECM-mimicking scaffolds manipulating the host immune response and FBR that are applied in the clinics [19].

2.2.3 Zwitterionic Biomaterials for Immunomodulation

Low-fouling zwitterionic molecules are extensively utilized to modify the implanted biomaterial surfaces preventing long-term fibrosis and increasing the host acceptance. It is well known that "zwitterionic polymers" describes polymers that contain a set of opposite charged functional groups in the backbone of recurring units. *Yesilyurt* et al. demonstrated innovative surface functionalization of alginate based polymeric capsules using zwitterionic phosphorylcholine polymer thin films. Further, the coating reduced the FBR on implanted materials including alginate and polystyrene microbeads when implanted in C57BL/6 J mouse model [20]. Jiang et al. demonstrated PCBMA hydrogel implantation sub-Q in C57BL/6 mice showing minimum FBR, collagen deposition and inflammatory response compared to pHEMA, following 12 weeks of implantation [21]. Detailed mechanistic analysis confirmed blood-vessels development, macrophage recruitment and anti-inflammation around the PCBMA hydrogels compared to the pHEMA. Zhang and coworkers reported novel fabrication strategy using poly sulfobetaine methacrylate (PSB) and polydopamine (PDA) coating to cochlear implants (CI) [22]. The coating with this zwitterionic polymer has increased the hydrophilicity, lower protein and cellular attachment, improved biocompatibility, and long-lasting durability to the implants in rat model preventing damage of CI implants and protecting from severe sensorineural hearing loss. Mechanistic studies revealed PSB-PDA coating to CI implants reduces the secretion of pro-inflammatory factors (IL-1β, TNF-α, NO) and pro-fibrotic factors (α-SMA, TGF-β1, collagen I) compared to the uncoated control implants, indicating the role PSB-PDA to mitigate fibrosis improving the treatments of CI. In another interesting work, *Asiyeh*

Golabchi et al., showed similar PSB-PDA coating strategy for neural electrode devices, reducing protein absorption, fibroblast adhesion, inflammation resulting in the prevention of fibrosis to the silicon based neural probes following implantation into mouse brain [23]. These discoveries prove the effective use of anti-fouling zwitterionic coating in the reduction of acute inflammation to the brain tissue following neural implants. Another pioneer work by Daniel G. Anderson and coworkers from the Massachusetts Institute of Technology (MIT), USA reported a combinatorial chemical approach to utilize coating of 64 different zwitterionic polymers improving the functions of continuous blood glucose monitors (CGM) [24]. Poly (MPC) coated sensors caused minimum fibrosis, had lowest inflammation, and improved the CGM applications when tested in the healthy and diabetic non-human primates. These recent results using zwitterionic coating to mitigate fibrosis are really encouraging. However, these coatings have a relatively weak mechanically, resulting in their inability to prevent long-term fibrosis around the medical implants.

2.3 Impact of Biomaterial's Physical Properties on Immunomodulation

Various design parameters of the medical implants and biomaterials including surface topography, size, shape and geometry, surface morphology, surface wettability, phenotype, mechanical stability, roughness, hydrophilicity/hydrophobicity, stiffness, site of implantation and porosity plays a crucial role in the response of the implants to FBR and host acceptance. These broad ranges of physical properties have a tremendous role in coordinating several biological properties including inhibiting FBR, protein corona attachment, macrophage adhesion and activation, in reaction to any foreign implanted materials. In this book chapter, we will mainly focus on the effect of surface topography, effect of surface geometry and mechanical stability and their roles in FBR.

2.3.1 Effect of Surface Topography on Immunomodulation

The surface structure of an implanted biomaterial has notable role manipulating the surrounding immune recognition, foreign body responses and host acceptance. It is well researched that smooth biomaterials surface-based implants including metal implants (titanium) are less prone to inflammation, macrophage recognition and fibrosis enhancing their durability and lifetime [9]. Changing the surface topography, roughness, charge, mechanical stability, and hydrophilicity/hydrophobicity play a major role affecting the immunogenicity of the implanted biomaterials affecting their outcomes against FBR. Further, protein adsorption along with resulting immune mechanistic cascades can be manipulated by changing the surface properties of the implanted biomaterials. McWhorter and coworkers showed the changes in macrophage attachment with the variation of various topographical parameters including structures, shapes and inclinations. They reported that modulation of micro-patterns can result in higher upregulation of M2-macrophage markers and reduced amount of proinflammatory cytokines resulting in the host acceptance and negligible FBR [25]. *Chen* et al. reported the influence of topography of biomaterials surface with the macrophage-associated fibrosis when gratings (500 nm to 2 mm parallel) used as a printed form on polymeric surface [26]. Higher the size of the gratings imprinted on the polymer implants, more the attachment of immune cells to the polymer surface. This significantly can impact the outcome of the implants in terms of host acceptance and durability. In general, metal-based titanium implants are less prone to macrophage attachments and immune recognition owing to their smooth metallic surface. However, activation of downstream inflammatory cascade can still impact in the implant failure in long-term.

In a recent published report by Robert Langer and colleagues, they demonstrated the role of the surface topography of silicone-based breast implants in the outcome of FBR, immune recognition and host-acceptance when these are tested in various in vivo model including rodents, rabbits, and human (Fig. 2.4) [27]. Silicone is broadly utilized for various medical implant applications due to its higher biocompatibility and long-durability. But, textured and rough surface of the silicone breast implants can cause macrophage adhesion resulting immune recognition, activation of pro-inflammatory cascades and other complications such as malignancies. The authors thoroughly tested various commercially approved silicone breast implants (average roughness, 0–90 μm) against their FBR when implanted in the mammary fat pads of either humans, rabbits, or rodents. The results showed the surface roughness and topography largely play an important role for the resulting immune response and host acceptance. An average roughness of 4 μm greatly reduced inflammation, FBR and long-term fibrosis when tested in in vivo models. Moreover, mechanistic studies showed involvement of immunosuppressor role of FOXP3 + regulatory T cells in the reduction of fibrosis around the implants. Manipulation of implant surfaces to increase the hydrophilicity or smoothness is an incredible strategy to mitigate fibrosis and reduce inflammatory cascades. In another published work, Alfarsi et al. fabricated acid-etched stereolithography (SLA) assisted implants with high hydrophilicity showing minimum pro-inflammatory response and FBR potentially increasing the host acceptance and durability of the implants [28]. Vassey and coworkers performed a high-throughput screening to test various micropillar assemblies of 2176 micropatterns in the macrophage adhesion and consequent inflammatory responses of the implants [29]. It was observed that micropillar size and density played a crucial role manipulating the fate of the immunogenic and inflammatory responses by altering the cell types from pro-inflammatory to anti-inflammatory state. Surfaces with micropillar diameter of 5–10 μm diameter had least macrophage adhesion and FBR compared to the other surfaces. By increasing the textures of the implant surface, creation of air pockets inside the surface ridges were reported that has created an elevated hydrophobicity. Moreover, surface patterning can dramatically change the protein adsorption and macrophage attachment resulting in the success of the implants with long durability. Real tissue like patterning can significantly improve the success of the implants by reducing the host immune response and mitigating FBR. Surface topography also assist in the regulation of the immune cascade reactions and manipulating the immune cell phenotypes towards the osteogenic developments at alloplastic planes [30].

2.3.2 Impact of the Implant Geometry on Immunomodulation

The effect of the geometry of implanted biomaterial including size and shape has an important role in affecting the FBR and host-acceptance [31–33]. Ward and coworkers demonstrated shape dependent effects of various biomaterials towards FBR. They showed that micro cylinders engineered out of several materials had wide scale of FBR dependent on the porosity and diameter of the cylinder. They performed in vivo studies on Sprague–Dawley rats and implanted those biomaterials for 7 weeks. Results showed that 0.3 mm diameter cylinders exhibited minimum fibrosis and lower capsule formation around the implant, whereas the bigger diameter cylinders (2 mm) showed pro-inflammation, higher FBR and a thick capsule formation around the implants. *Salthouse* et al., performed detailed animal studies using various medical grade rods with different cross-sections and determine their biocompatibility and FBR [31]. Interestingly, minimum fibrosis was found with the rods having circular patterning compared to other patterned cross sections (pentagonal or triangular). Recent several studies confirmed that non-textured biomaterials implant surface showed that smooth surfaced material elicits less acute immune reactions than implants with sharp ends and acute angles. Veiseh and coworkers showed role of size and geometry of the implanted biomaterials with FBR and host acceptance, modulating the long-term biocompatibility [32]. A large screening of various diameter (0.3–1.9 mm) sized hydrogel capsules in rodents confirmed minimum FBR in capsules of size over 1.5 mm, whereas microcapsules of size less than 0.5 mm triggered severe FBR and fibrosis around them (Fig. 2.5). Eight distinct sized (0.3, 0.4, 0.5, 0.6, 0.7, 1, 1.5, and 1.9 mm) capsules were implanted to the intraperitoneal space of immunocompetent C57BL/6 mice for two weeks. Following two weeks retrieval, the capsules were analyzed using dark-field and bright-field microscopy to assess the degree of fibrosis and collagen deposition. The results showed notable reduction of fibrosis deposition with increase in capsules size indicating role of geometry with FBR and host immune response. Similar observation was there when implants were made of diverse range of materials including glass, plastic, metal etc. This indicated that the effect on FBR is primarily due to the implant geometry such as size and less on surface area or the nature of the implanted materials. In another interesting publication the author demonstrated the effects of implant size on macrophage adhesion, inflammation and FBR. Various sized titanium nanorods were implanted and results demonstrated minimum FBR in implants of size 60–70 nm [33].

2 Immunomodulation Strategies Using Biomaterial Chemistry ...

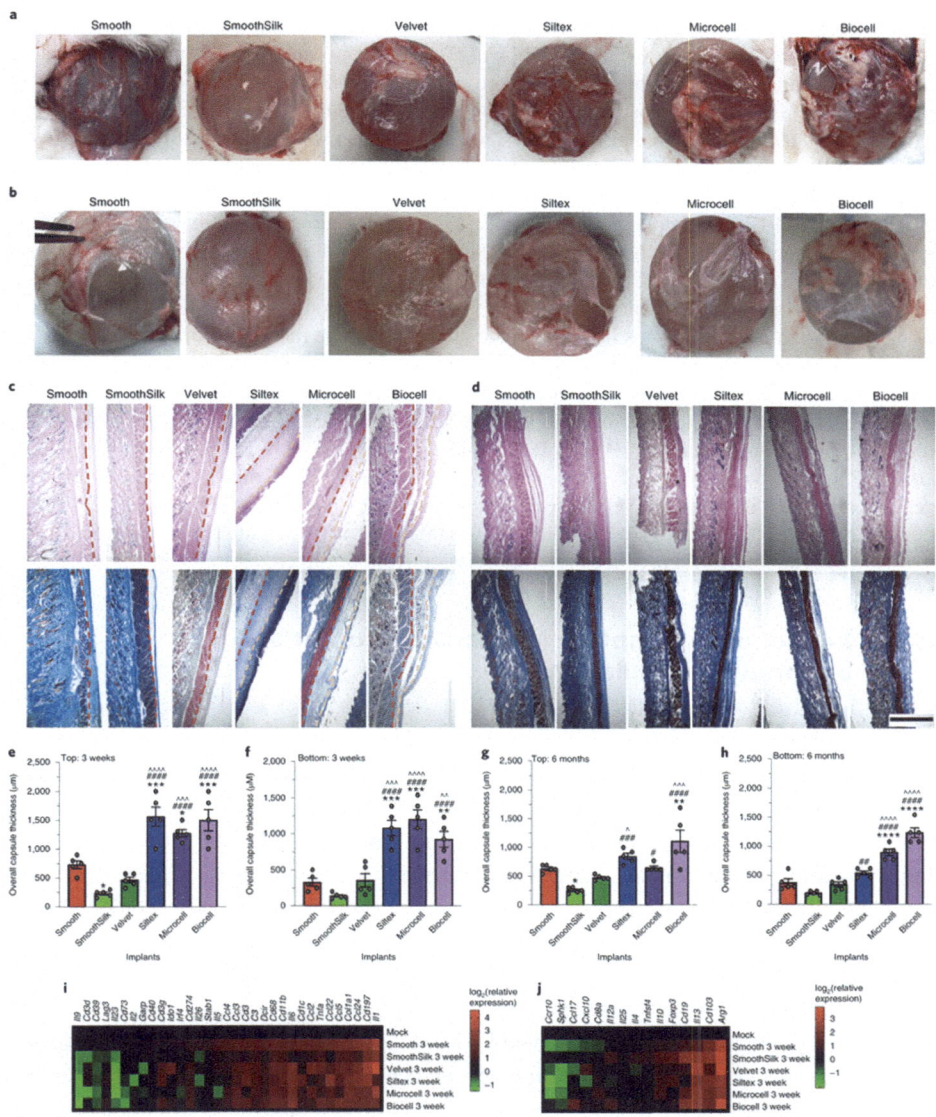

◄**Fig. 2.4** Breast implant surface topography affects host response and fibrosis in rabbits a,b, Human-scale (205 cm^3) breast implants explanted following 3 week **a** or 6 month **b** subcutaneous implantations in New Zealand White rabbits. **c, d**, H&E (top) and Masson's trichrome (bottom)-stained histologic sections of tissue and capsules surrounding 3 week **c** and 6 month **d** subcutaneous implants. Scale bar, 1,000 µm; original magnification, × 4. **e, f**, Fibrotic capsule thickness surrounding 3 week implants on their top subcutaneous side **e** or bottom (deeper tissue) side **f**. **g, h**, Six-month top **g** and bottom **h** capsule thickness. Double capsules were observed as early as three weeks for Siltex, Microcell and Biocell implants, with strong Velcro effects upon dissection and separation of implant and tissue capsule for histology processing (Supplementary Videos 1–3). Five measurements of capsule thickness were taken for 5 different fields of view from 2 different regions of tissue, with numbers then compiled across n = 5 rabbits per group. i, j, Nano String analysis of 3 week human-scale subcutaneous implants in New Zealand White rabbits for immune markers and cytokines, compared with mock (saline-injected) controls. Patterns of downregulation **i** and upregulation **j** in the Smooth Silk group suggests differential immune modulation. In bar graphs, data are mean ± s.e.m. of biological replicates. One-way analysis of variance (ANOVA) plus Bonferroni multiple-comparisons correction; ***$P < 0.001$ and ****$P < 0.0001$ versus control; ###$P < 0.001$ and ####$P < 0.0001$ versus Smooth Silk; and ^^^$P < 0.001$ and ^^^^$P < 0.0001$ versus Velvet Surface. *$P = 0.0418$ (Smooth Silk versus control) and 0.0237 (Microcell versus control) (e); **$P = 0.002$ and ^^$P = 0.0031$ (f); *$P = 0.0418$, **$P = 0.0058$, #$P = 0.0314$ and ^$P = 0.0458$ (g); ##$P = 0.0019$ (h). The figure is reproduced after permission from Springer Nature [27]

2.3.3 Impact of the Implant Mechanical Properties on Immunomodulation

The mechanical characteristics of a biomaterial play crucial role for varying biological responses including inflammatory signals and FBR. Mechanical properties of the biomaterial such as displacements and functional loads influence the reaction of it under separate force structures, resulting in strains and stresses [34]. The biomaterials containing insufficient mechanical stability and strength were unable to support for tissue growth and regeneration properties. However, over-rigid materials also impede tissue reinforcement, and henceforth an imbalance of mechanical properties can be detrimental for mitigating FBR and host acceptance. Various studies were performed to demonstrate that the mechanical properties of the implanted biomaterials has a significant role on the macrophage attachment and associated M1/M2 polarization cascades that influence the host immune response and implant acceptance [35, 36]. It has been shown that rigid materials promote M1 macrophage polarization or associated pro-inflammatory cascades whereas, soft-implants instigate M1-macrophage polarization or anti-inflammatory responses. The modulation of the mechanical stiffness of the 3D-implants made of polyethylene glycol-RGD enhances the anti-inflammatory responses due to low rigidity of the material mitigating FBR and fibrosis. Mixed rigid cues with sodium alginate hydrogels and bioactive glass reduces the implant stiffness promoting anti-inflammatory responses and skin repair.

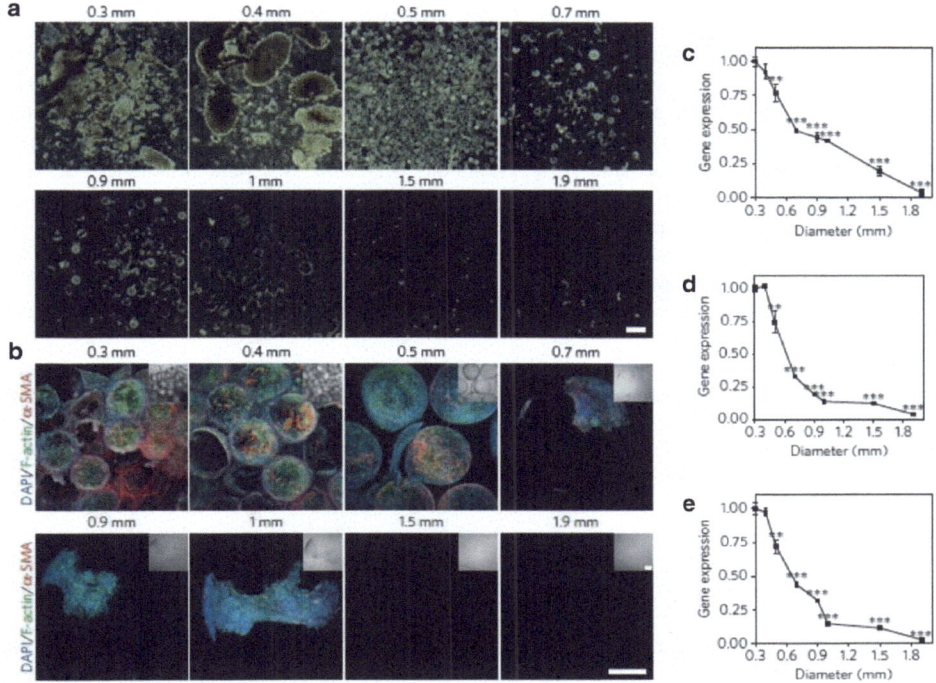

Fig. 2.5 Increasing alginate sphere size results in reduced cellular deposition and fibrosis formation on the spheres. SLG20 alginate spheres (0.5 ml in volume) of eight different sizes (0.3, 0.4, 0.5, 0.6, 0.7, 1, 1.5, and 1.9 mm) were implanted into the intraperitoneal space of C57BL/6 mice, where they were retained for 14 days and analyzed for degree of fibrosis on retrieval. **a** Dark-field phase-contrast images obtained from retrieved spheres reveal a significant decrease in the level of cellular overgrowth with an increase in sphere size. Scale bar, 2 mm. **b** Z-stacked confocal images of retrieved spheres immunofluorescence stained with DAPI (highlighting cellular nuclei), phalloidin (highlighting F-actin), and α-SMA (highlighting myofibroblast cells). Scale bar, 300 m. **c–e**, qPCR-based expression analysis of fibrotic markers α-SMA **c**, Collagen 1a1 (**d**, Col1a1) and Collagen 1a2 (**e**, Col1a2) directly on the eight different sphere sizes (0.3, 0.4, 0.5, 0.7, 0.9, 1, 1.5 and 1.9 mm) plotted normalized to relative expression levels on 300-m spheres. The figure and caption are reproduced after permission from Spring Nature, 2015 [32])

References

1. Mariani, E., Lisignoli, G., Borzì, R.M. and Pulsatelli, L., 2019. Biomaterials: foreign bodies or tuners for the immune response?. *International journal of molecular sciences*, 20(3), p.636.
2. Capuani, S., Malgir, G., Chua, C.Y.X. and Grattoni, A., 2022. Advanced strategies to thwart foreign body response to implantable devices. *Bioengineering & Translational Medicine*, 7(3), p.e10300.

3. Cravedi, P., Farouk, S., Angeletti, A., Edgar, L., Tamburrini, R., Duisit, J., Perin, L. and Orlando, G., 2017. Regenerative immunology: the immunological reaction to biomaterials. *Transplant International*, *30*(12), pp.1199-1208.
4. Taraballi, F., Sushnitha, M., Tsao, C., Bauza, G., Liverani, C., Shi, A. and Tasciotti, E., 2018. Biomimetic tissue engineering: tuning the immune and inflammatory response to implantable biomaterials. *Advanced healthcare materials*, *7*(17), p.1800490.
5. Kim, B., Pradhan, L., Hernandez, A., Yenurkar, D., Nethi, S.K. and Mukherjee, S., Current Advances in Immunomodulatory Biomaterials for Cell Therapy and Tissue Engineering. Advanced Therapeutics, p. 2300002.
6. Bridges, A.W., Singh, N., Burns, K.L., Babensee, J.E., Lyon, L.A. and García, A.J., 2008. Reduced acute inflammatory responses to microgel conformal coatings. *Biomaterials*, *29*(35), pp.4605–4615. [7] T. Wong, S. Kang, S. Tang, E. Smythe, B. Hatton, A. Grinthal, J. Aizenberg, *Nature*. **2011**, *477*, 443
7. Lin, C.C., Metters, A.T. and Anseth, K.S., 2009. Functional PEG–peptide hydrogels to modulate local inflammation induced by the pro-inflammatory cytokine TNFα. *Biomaterials*, *30*(28), pp.4907-4914.
8. Vegas, A.J., Veiseh, O., Doloff, J.C., Ma, M., Tam, H.H., Bratlie, K., Li, J., Bader, A.R., Langan, E., Olejnik, K. and Fenton, P., 2016. Combinatorial hydrogel library enables identification of materials that mitigate the foreign body response in primates. *Nature biotechnology*, *34*(3), pp.345-352.
9. Sanchez-Cano, C. and Carril, M., 2020. Recent developments in the design of non-biofouling coatings for nanoparticles and surfaces. *International Journal of Molecular Sciences*, *21*(3), p.1007.
10. Mukherjee, S., Kim, B., Cheng, L.Y., Doerfert, M.D., Li, J., Hernandez, A., Liang, L., Jarvis, M.I., Rios, P.D., Ghani, S. and Joshi, I., 2023. Screening hydrogels for antifibrotic properties by implanting cellularly barcoded alginates in mice and a non-human primate. *Nature Biomedical Engineering*, 7, (2023), pages 867–886.
11. Karinja, S.J., Bernstein, J.L., Mukherjee, S., Jin, J., Lin, A., Abadeer, A., Kaymakcalan, O., Veiseh, O. and Spector, J.A., 2023. An Anti-Fibrotic Breast Implant Surface Coating Significantly Reduces Peri-Prosthetic Capsule Formation. Plastic and Reconstructive Surgery, p. e010323.
12. Wright, M.A., Miller, A.J., Dong, X., Karinja, S.J., Samadi, A., Lara, D.O., Mukherjee, S., Veiseh, O. and Spector, J.A., 2023. Reducing Peri-Implant Capsule Thickness in Submuscular Rodent Model of Breast Reconstruction with Delayed Radiotherapy. Journal of Surgical Research, 291, pp.158-166.
13. Rostam, H.M., Fisher, L.E., Hook, A.L., Burroughs, L., Luckett, J.C., Figueredo, G.P., Mbadugha, C., Teo, A.C., Latif, A., Kämmerling, L. and Day, M., 2020. Immune-instructive polymers control macrophage phenotype and modulate the foreign body response in vivo. Matter, 2(6), pp.1564-1581.
14. Alobaid, M.A., Richards, S.J., Alexander, M.R., Gibson, M.I. and Ghaemmaghami, A.M., 2020. Developing immune-regulatory materials using immobilized monosaccharides with immuneinstructive properties. Materials Today Bio, 8, p.100080.
15. Kou, P.M., Pallassana, N., Bowden, R., Cunningham, B., Joy, A., Kohn, J. and Babensee, J.E., 2012. Predicting biomaterial property-dendritic cell phenotype relationships from the multivariate analysis of responses to polymethacrylates. *Biomaterials*, *33*(6), pp.1699-1713.
16. Kajahn, J., Franz, S., Rueckert, E., Forstreuter, I., Hintze, V., Moeller, S. and Simon, J.C., 2012. Artificial extracellular matrices composed of collagen I and high sulfated hyaluronan modulate monocyte to macrophage differentiation under conditions of sterile inflammation. *Biomatter*, *2*(4), pp.226-273.

17. Brown, B.N., Londono, R., Tottey, S., Zhang, L., Kukla, K.A., Wolf, M.T., Daly, K.A., Reing, J.E. and Badylak, S.F., 2012. Macrophage phenotype as a predictor of constructive remodeling following the implantation of biologically derived surgical mesh materials [Acta Biomaterialia 8 (2012) 978–987]. *Acta biomaterialia*, *8*(7), p.2871.
18. Dziki, J.L., Huleihel, L., Scarritt, M.E. and Badylak, S.F., 2017. Extracellular matrix bioscaffolds as immunomodulatory biomaterials. *Tissue Engineering Part A*, *23*(19-20), pp.1152-1159.
19. Yesilyurt, V., Veiseh, O., Doloff, J.C., Li, J., Bose, S., Xie, X., Bader, A.R., Chen, M., Webber, M.J., Vegas, A.J. and Langer, R., 2017. A facile and versatile method to endow biomaterial devices with zwitterionic surface coatings. Advanced healthcare materials, 6(4), p.1601091.
20. Jiang, S. and Cao, Z., 2010. Ultralow-fouling, functionalizable, and hydrolyzable zwitterionic materials and their derivatives for biological applications. *Advanced materials*, *22*(9), pp.920-932.
21. Chen, A., Chen, D., Lv, K., Li, G., Pan, J., Ma, D., Tang, J. and Zhang, H., 2023. Zwitterionic polymer/polydopamine coating of electrode arrays reduces fibrosis and residual hearing loss after cochlear implantation. Advanced Healthcare Materials, 12(1), p.2200807.
22. Golabchi, A., Wu, B., Cao, B., Bettinger, C.J. and Cui, X.T., 2019. Zwitterionic polymer/polydopamine coating reduce acute inflammatory tissue responses to neural implants. Biomaterials, 225, p.119519.
23. X Xie, J. Doloff1, V. Yesilyurt, A. Sadraei, J. McGarrigle, M. Omami, O. Veiseh, S. Farah, D. Isa, S. Ghani, I. Joshi, A. Vegas, J. Li, W. Wang, A. Bader, H. Tam, J. Tao, H. Chen, B. Yang, K. Williamson, J. Oberholzer, R. Langer, D. Anderson, Nat Biomed Eng., 2018, 2, 894.
24. McWhorter, F.Y., Wang, T., Nguyen, P., Chung, T. and Liu, W.F., 2013. Modulation of macrophage phenotype by cell shape. *Proceedings of the National Academy of Sciences*, *110*(43), pp.17253-17258.
25. Chen, S., Jones, J.A., Xu, Y., Low, H.Y., Anderson, J.M. and Leong, K.W., 2010. Characterization of topographical effects on macrophage behavior in a foreign body response model. Biomaterials, 31(13), pp.3479-3491.
26. Doloff, J.C., Veiseh, O., de Mezerville, R., Sforza, M., Perry, T.A., Haupt, J., Jamiel, M., Chambers, C., Nash, A., Aghlara-Fotovat, S. and Stelzel, J.L., 2021. The surface topography of silicone breast implants mediates the foreign body response in mice, rabbits and humans. Nature biomedical engineering, 5(10), pp.1115-1130.
27. Alfarsi, M.A., Hamlet, S.M. and Ivanovski, S., 2014. Titanium surface hydrophilicity modulates the human macrophage inflammatory cytokine response. *Journal of Biomedical Materials Research Part A: An Official Journal of The Society for Biomaterials, The Japanese Society for Biomaterials, and The Australian Society for Biomaterials and the Korean Society for Biomaterials*, *102*(1), pp.60-67.
28. Vassey, M.J., Figueredo, G.P., Scurr, D.J., Vasilevich, A.S., Vermeulen, S., Carlier, A., Luckett, J., Beijer, N.R., Williams, P., Winkler, D.A. and de Boer, J., 2020. Immune modulation by design: using topography to control human monocyte attachment and macrophage differentiation. *Advanced Science*, *7*(11), p. 1903392. [30] S. Shirazi, S. Ravindran, L. Cooper biomaterial., 2022, 291, 121903.
29. Matlaga, B.F., Yasenchak, L.P. and Salthouse, T.N., 1976. Tissue response to implanted polymers: the significance of sample shape. *Journal of biomedical materials research*, *10*(3), pp.391-397.
30. O. Veiseh, J. Doloff, M. Ma, A. Vegas, H. Tam, A. Bader, J. Li, E. Langan, J. Wyckoff, W. Loo, S. Jhunjhunwala, A. Chiu, S. Siebert, K. Tang, J. Lock, S. Dasilva, M. Bochenek, J. Elias, Y. Wang, M. Qi, D. Lavin, M. Chen, N. Dholakia, R. Thakrar, I Lacík, G. Weir, J. Oberholzer, D. Greiner, R. Langer, D. Anderson. Nat Mater., 2015, 14, 643.

31. Rajyalakshmi, A., Ercan, B., Balasubramanian, K. and Webster, T.J., 2011. Reduced adhesion of macrophages on anodized titanium with select nanotube surface features. *International journal of nanomedicine*, pp. 1765–1771.
32. Wang, L., Wang, C., Wu, S., Fan, Y. and Li, X., 2020. Influence of the mechanical properties of biomaterials on degradability, cell behaviors and signaling pathways: current progress and challenges. *Biomaterials science*, 8(10), pp.2714-2733.
33. Guimarães, C.F., Gasperini, L., Marques, A.P. and Reis, R.L., 2020. The stiffness of living tissues and its implications for tissue engineering. *Nature Reviews Materials*, 5(5), pp.351-370.
34. Atcha, A. Jairaman, J. Holt, V. Meli, R. Nagalla, P. Veerasubramanian, K. Brumm, H. Lim, S. Othy, M. Cahalan, M. Pathak, W. Liu, Nat Commun., 2021, 12, 3256.
35. Blakney, A.K., Swartzlander, M.D. and Bryant, S.J., 2012. The effects of substrate stiffness on the in vitro activation of macrophages and in vivo host response to poly (ethylene glycol)-based hydrogels. *Journal of biomedical materials research. Part A*, 100(6), p.1375.
36. Zhu, Y., Deng, S., Ma, Z., Kong, L., Li, H. and Chan, H.F., 2021. Macrophages activated by akermanite/alginate composite hydrogel stimulate migration of bone marrow-derived mesenchymal stem cells. *Biomedical Materials*, 16(4), p.045004.

Use of Immunomodulatory Biomaterials in Diabetes Therapy

Boram Kim and Sudip Mukherjee

3.1 Introduction

Type 1 diabetes is a complex and chronic autoimmune disease that affects millions of individuals worldwide. It is characterized by the destruction of insulin-producing β-cells in the pancreas, leading to a deficiency of insulin and subsequent high blood sugar levels [1–3]. Although the precise triggers remain elusive, it is widely believed that a combination of genetic predisposition and environmental triggers, such as viral infections, initiate an autoimmune response, leading to the destruction of pancreatic β-cells [5]. This autoimmune attack disrupts the production of insulin. As insulin is responsible for regulating glucose levels in the blood, the absence of insulin leads to an accumulation of glucose in the bloodstream, causing hyperglycemia. As T1D progresses, it gives rise to a multitude of complications that can significantly impact an individual's health and well-being. This can result in various symptoms such as increased thirst, frequent urination, unexplained weight loss, fatigue, and blurred vision [3, 5]. The incidence of T1D varies between countries and populations. On average, it is estimated that around 1 in 300 to 1 in 500 children and adolescents worldwide develop T1D each year. T1D represents 5–10% of the diagnosed cases of diabetes, corresponding to more than 1.8 million individuals in the United States and 20 million worldwide [1]. Exogenous insulin injections are the most common treatment to delay the onset and reduce the progression of diabetic complications. Even

B. Kim
Department of Bioengineering, Rice University Houston, TX, USA

S. Mukherjee (✉)
School of Biomedical Engineering, Indian Institute of Technology (BHU), Varanasi 221005, UP, India
e-mail: sudip.bme@iitbhu.ac.in

with advances in the development of long-lasting insulin and insulin pumps, they do not perfectly simulate insulin secretion from pancreatic β-cells, and a patient's blood glucose levels fluctuate despite close monitoring and frequent adjustments of insulin does [1, 9, 10]. In addition, insulin therapy can cause patients to experience life-threatening hypoglycemic (suppressed blood glucose below normal levels) unawareness, a dangerous acute complication caused by delayed insulin action. Furthermore, long-term glucose imbalance can result in hyperglycemia-related to microvascular and macrovascular complications [1, 11]. According to statistics, patients with T1D have a much higher risk of cardiovascular disease than people without T1D, and approximately 30% of T1D patients are diagnosed with chronic kidney disease [12]. This is the primary rationale for many groups to design therapies to provide the diabetic patient with an endogenous insulin source that regulates blood glucose on a natural, minute-to-minute basis [10].

3.2 Conventional Therapies in Diabetes and Limitations

Pancreas and islet transplantation are potential treatments for T1D, particularly for those with severe complications or difficulty managing blood sugar levels despite insulin therapy. Whole pancreas transplantation involves replacing the entire pancreas, including the cells that produce insulin, with a healthy pancreas from a donor. Pancreas transplantation can restore insulin production, eliminate the need for insulin injections, and improve blood sugar control. A successful pancreas transplant provides almost normal glucose homeostasis, but it requires life-long immunosuppressive medication and is associated with major surgery and high morbidity [1, 10]. Since it is still unclear whether the benefits of a pancreas transplant over continued insulin treatment outweigh the disadvantages, most transplant centers still restrict themselves to combined pancreas and kidney transplantation in diabetic patients with end-stage renal failure [10, 13].

Pancreatic islet transplantation involves transplanting the cells in the pancreas that produce insulin, called islets, into the recipient's liver. The islets are harvested from a donor pancreas and purified before transplantation. In contrast to pancreas transplantation, islet transplantation requires no major surgery. Transplantation of human islets into the portal vein (Edmonton protocol, Fig. 3.1) has demonstrated success among patients, with many sustaining normoglycemia for three to five years after transplantation, with 10% sustaining normoglycemia for more than five years [12].

Islet transplantation is beneficial for individuals with T1D as it restores glycemic control and enhances their quality of life [14]. However, there are significant challenges that hinder its widespread use. A key issue is the requirement for continuous immunosuppression to prevent rejection of the transplanted tissue, coupled with a shortage of available pancreas donors [15]. Additionally, approximately 60% of transplanted islets are destroyed by the immediate inflammatory response from the blood, leaving a small remaining β-cell mass at risk of metabolic exhaustion, hypoxic damage, and immune

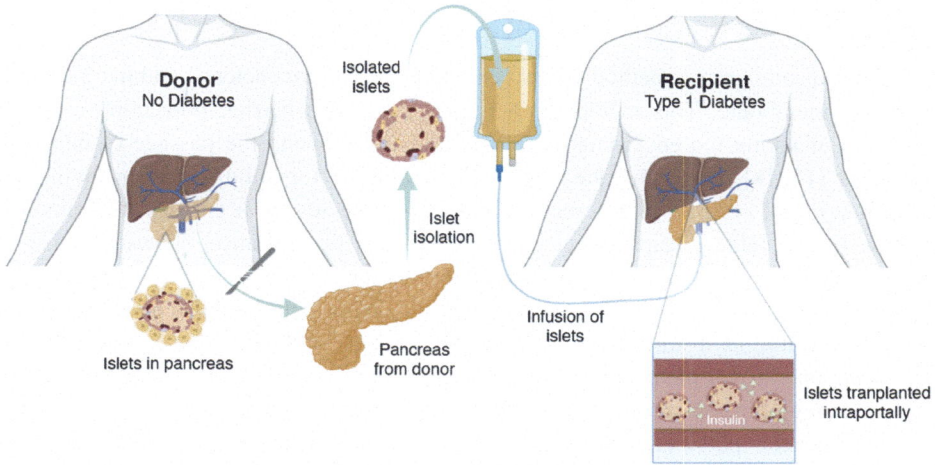

Fig. 3.1 Edmonton protocol for Islets transplantation. Figure is made using Biorender.com

rejection [16]. Moreover, the immune system's harmful attack on the transplanted cells leads to long-term graft failure, necessitating multiple islet transplantations to achieve sustained control of blood glucose levels (>10,000 IEQ/kg recipient body weight) [16] (Table 3.1).

3.3 Cell Therapies for Diabetes and Their Challenges

There are several sources of β-cells that can be used for transplantation for T1D treatment. Cadaveric pancreatic islets isolated from donors are the most common source of β-cells transplantation. These islets are purified and transplanted into the recipient's liver, where they can start producing insulin. However, the supply of donor islets is limited, and there is a high risk of rejection. As an unlimited supply of β-cells for transplantation, two strategies have been investigated. Stem cell-derived β-cells are the potential source, which can differentiate into β-cells in the laboratory. This approach has the potential to produce an unlimited supply of β-cells, but more research is needed to optimize the differentiation process and ensure the safety of the cells. For example, human embryonic stem cell (hESC)-derived β-cells often contain undifferentiated stem cells, which may pose some regulatory concerns regarding teratoma formation [1, 11, 17]. Xenogeneic β-cells can also be harvested from animals, such as pigs, and transplanted into humans. However, this approach raises concerns about immune rejection and the transmission of animal viruses to humans [11, 17]. Xenogeneic tissue induces potent rejection responses that cannot be safely and effectively controlled by anti-rejection medicine [5]. Therefore, researchers are exploring ways to protect β-cells from immune attacks, such as encapsulating them in biomaterials that prevent immune cells from accessing the cells while allowing insulin to be secreted.

Cell encapsulation is a method where cells, like β-cells, are enclosed within a partially permeable membrane. This membrane acts as a protective barrier, preventing immune cells from attacking the encapsulated cells while still allowing the passage of nutrients and insulin [11, 18]. This technique is particularly valuable for cell therapies involving the transplantation of cells from different individuals or species, as it enables the immuno-isolation of the cells. Encapsulating pancreatic β-cells, for instance, shows promise in treating diabetes by addressing issues like donor shortages and the need for immunosuppression. The primary objective of an encapsulation device is to establish an environment that facilitates normal insulin secretion in response to varying blood glucose levels. It also ensures the viability of the encapsulated cells by shielding them from the immune system and facilitating efficient exchange of nutrients and waste products [17, 19].

Among several polymeric materials, seaweed-derived linear polysaccharide alginate has been extensively studied as a desirable candidate for cell encapsulation. Alginate converts into a gel form by ionic cross-linking with bivalent cations [2]. Alginate has several properties that make it attractive for cell encapsulation. First, alginate is a biocompatible material, meaning it does not elicit an immune response when implanted in the body. This makes it suitable for use in cell therapy applications. Second, alginate can form a semi-permeable membrane around cells, which allows for the diffusion of small molecules, such as nutrients and oxygen, while preventing the diffusion of larger molecules, such as antibodies and immune cells. This can protect the encapsulated cells from immune attack. Also, alginate can form a hydrogel with a range of mechanical properties, depending on the concentration and molecular weight of the alginate used. This allows for the creation of alginate beads or capsules with varying degrees of stiffness or elasticity, which can be tailored to different cell therapy applications [2, 13, 20]. In addition, alginate is stable under a wide range of conditions, including physiological conditions, making it suitable for long-term implantation in the body. Alginate has been used for cell encapsulation in a variety of cell therapy applications, including islet transplantation for the treatment of diabetes, as well as for encapsulating other types of cells, such as neural stem cells and mesenchymal stem cells [2, 13, 20]. In 1980, Lim and Sun conducted a study where they utilized microcapsules made of alginate to treat diabetes in rats [21]. Their findings demonstrated extended survival of islet grafts compared to free islets. The encapsulated islets were able to survive for up to 3 weeks, whereas the free islets only survived for 8 days without the use of immunosuppression [2, 13, 20]. However, the graft eventually failed within a few weeks due to the microcapsule's limited biocompatibility and the host immune cells' foreign body response. Over time, the formation of a fibrous capsule around the alginate beads hindered the diffusion of nutrients and oxygen to the encapsulated cells. Ongoing research is focused on optimizing alginate encapsulation techniques to enhance the survival and functionality of the encapsulated cells.

3.4 Graft Failure

As previously mentioned, one of the major challenges in the clinical application of cell encapsulation is the limited availability of suitable biomaterials. The materials used for cell encapsulation have shown immunogenic properties, resulting in the formation of tissue capsules and subsequent failure of the cell graft [22, 23]. When implanted, these biomaterials trigger foreign body responses (FBR), which involve inflammatory events, wound-healing processes, and ultimately fibrosis, leading to the failure of the implanted device [24]. For instance, unmodified cell-free alginate, even in a small number of transplants, can induce FBR through immune recognition. Encapsulating allogeneic or xenogeneic donor tissue can further enhance this fibrotic response [2]. The aggregation of capsules and fibrosis around the biomaterial obstructs nutrient access to the cells, contributing to the decline in cell viability and function [25].

Additionally, there is a suggestion that encapsulated cells can be detected by the host adaptive immune system through an indirect antigen recognition pathway [4]. In general, host immune cells recognize foreign antigens through two pathways: direct and indirect recognition. Direct recognition occurs when host T cells identify donor antigens on the surface of foreign cells via donor MHC molecules [26]. Indirect antigen recognition occurs when host antigen-presenting cells (APCs) collect, and process antigens shed by the donor before presenting them to host T cells in an MHC-restricted manner [26, 27]. Regardless of the antigen presentation pathway, both result in the activation and expansion of graft-specific effector cells, which mediate the destruction of the foreign graft through cytotoxic CD8 + T cells and graft-specific antibody responses [4, 26]. Studies indicate that complete polymeric encapsulation can prevent direct antigen recognition by preventing direct contact between donor and host cells [28]. However, it is hypothesized that host immune recognition may still occur through indirect antigen recognition, as foreign shed antigens diffuse through the biomaterial and reach the peri-transplant site [4, 12] (Fig. 3.2).

3.5 Development of Immunomodulatory Biomaterials for Diabetes Therapy

It is crucial to discover novel immunomodulatory biomaterials that can serve as a carrier for β-cell transplantation to overcome clinical challenges. These materials should help reduce FBR, limit pericapsular fibrotic overgrowth, and improve the long-term viability and functionality of the graft cells. By customizing biomaterial design parameters, it is possible to generate specific and durable immunomodulation. Surface properties of biomaterials, such as topography, charge, and adhesive ligands, can be manipulated to induce desired immune cell phenotypes [29]. Recent studies have investigated modifying alginate hydrogel platforms to modulate immune responses and prevent fibrosis for islet

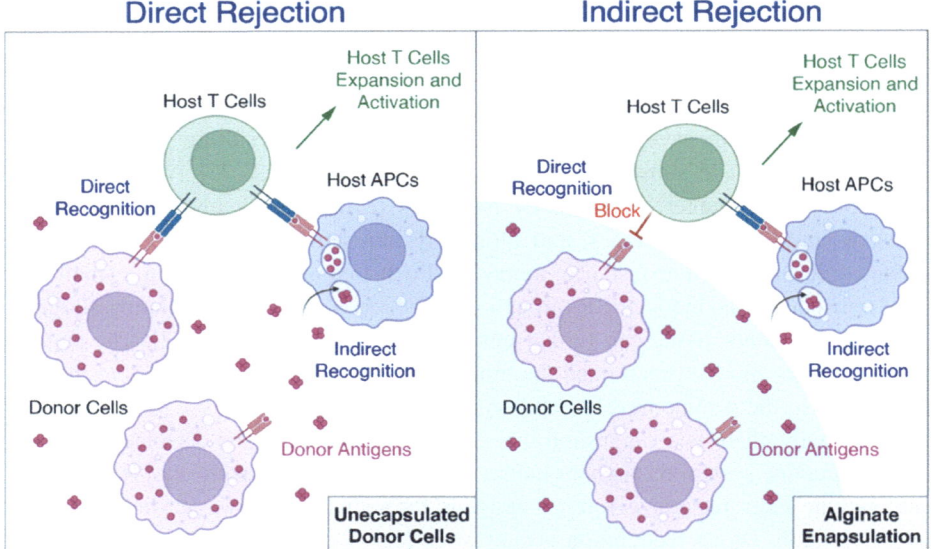

Fig. 3.2 Antigen Recognition Pathways of Unencapsulated and Microencapsulated Cells by the Host Adaptive Immune System. Figure is made using Biorender.com with concept adaptation from Li, et al. [4]

transplantation in different ways. First of all, the modifying structural design of encapsulation device can improve the functionality of device for long-term. Wang et al. devised a novel nanofibrous encapsulation device designed for the safe delivery of insulin-producing cells to effectively treat T1D [30]. The encapsulation device, composed of biocompatible nanofibers, offers an innovative approach to protect the transplanted insulin-producing cells from the immune system while allowing the diffusion of insulin and other essential nutrients. The study highlights the device's successful implementation in a preclinical trial involving animal models with induced diabetes. The encapsulated insulin-producing cells demonstrated long-term viability and functionality, leading to improved blood glucose regulation without the need for external insulin administration. Future studies and clinical trials are needed to validate these findings and determine the device's viability for human use.

In addition, chemically modifying alginate with zwitterionic groups reduced the cellular overgrowth of alginate capsules in different species and improved outcomes of islet encapsulation in a diabetic mouse model [31]. The researchers proposed that the modification of alginates with zwitterionic moieties can prevent the attachment and proliferation of unwanted cells on the surface of encapsulated cells, thereby improving the functionality and survival of the encapsulated cells. The study demonstrated that zwitterionically modified alginates effectively reduce cellular overgrowth when compared to unmodified alginates. Moreover, the modified alginates maintained their immunoprotective properties, allowing for the encapsulation of cells without compromising their function. Despite the promising results, the study primarily focused on fibroblast cells, and the effects of zwitterionically modified alginates on other cell types or complex cell systems remain to be explored. Additionally, the long-term stability and biocompatibility of the modified alginates need further investigation to ensure their suitability for clinical applications. In other study, researchers investigated a wide range of alginate analogs and found that making chemical modifications significantly reduced the fibrotic response in animal models [8, 32]. They observed that all the top analogs were modified with triazole derivatives, suggesting that the presence of triazoles on the material's surface might influence immune cell populations by deterring macrophage recognition [2, 15, 33]. Furthermore, the researchers utilized this lead material and delivered allogeneic pancreatic islets encapsulated in lead alginate to non-human primate model to access the efficacy of encapsulation materials [30] (Fig. 3.3). The study assessed the viability, functionality, and immune response to the encapsulated islet cells over an extended period. Furthermore, the study observed minimal signs of inflammation or foreign body response around the encapsulated islet cells, suggesting good biocompatibility and bio-integration of the alginate capsules within the omental bursa. Long-term graft survival and sustained islet function were achieved, indicating the potential of alginate encapsulation as a viable strategy for long-term immune protection in islet transplantation.

In a subsequent study, the researchers utilized these chemically modified alginates, particularly triazole-thiomorpholine dioxide alginate, to encapsulate human stem cell-derived beta cells (SC-β cells) and assessed their ability to control blood sugar levels in a diabetic animal model with a functioning immune system [34]. The authors demonstrated that alginate analogs with triazole modifications could reduce FBR, and SC-β cells encapsulated in these alginate hydrogels effectively maintained glucose responsiveness and long-term glycemic correction without the need for immuno-suppressive treatment. In 2023, Mukherjee and Kim et al. developed a second generation of library based on the previous triazole modification of alginate analogs [32] to find even better antifibrotic biomaterials with improved immunomodulatory functions [7]. The library of alginate analogs was screeded using a novel cellular barcoding strategy. Twenty unique human umbilical vein endothelial cells (HUVEC) from different donors were used as a barcode to tag each material's identity. The mixture of materials was implanted into intraperitoneal space, and the fibrosis outcomes 4 weeks postimplant were revealed by demultiplexing HUVEC genotypes and identifying the encapsulated donors. This method allowed the screening of 20 materials in a single rodent model and 100 materials in a non-human primate at once. The lead material showing an antifibrotic effect from this screening in mice study was used to deliver human islets in STZ-induced diabetic immunocompetent mice without immunosuppressive drugs. The islets encapsulated within lead alginate formulation showed long-term glycemic control for 80 days, while those within unmodified alginate failed to restore normal controls after 30 days postimplant (Fig. 3.4). Furthermore,

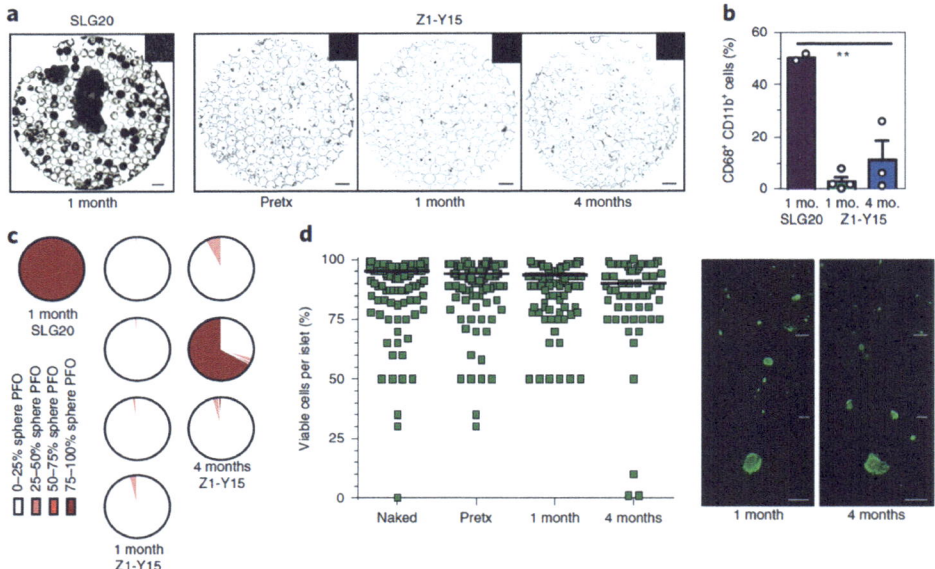

Fig. 3.3 Z1-Y15 alginate protects viable and glucose-responsive allogeneic islets in NHPs without any immunosuppression. **a** Representative inverted phase-contrast of retrieved spheres: SLG20 empty spheres at 1 month, Z1-Y15 spheres with encapsulated allogeneic islets pre-transplantation (pretx), post retrieval from NHPs at 1 month and 4 months (inserts are the non-inverted phase contrast images). Scale bars, 2 mm. **b** Percentages of CD68 + /CD11b + macrophage populations dissociated from retrieved sphere surfaces using flow cytometry. **c** Histograms depicting the degree of PFO sphere coverage for each of the primate retrievals at 1 month (SLG20 and Z1-Y15) and 4 months (Z1-Y15) post-transplantation in NHPs. White and light colours depict little sphere coverage by fibrosis and dark red shading depict spheres mostly fibrosed. **d** Left: estimated percentages of viable cells within islet cell clusters following live/dead staining performed pre-encapsulation (naked), post encapsulation in Z1-Y15 alginate (pretx) and post retrieval of non-fibrosed spheres at 1 month and 4 months. Right: representative fluorescent images of retrieved Z1-Y15 encapsulated allogeneic islets with the live/dead stains FDA and PI at 1 month and 4 months. Scale bars, 0.5 mm (top and middle); 0.2 mm (bottom). Reproduced with permission [8]. Copyright 2018, Springer Nature

this lead material was able to maintain blood glucose levels even with highly packed islet density within capsules. This result shows promising potential for applying a small medical device to prevent fibrosis and protect islets long-term with a high dose of islet transplantation.

Another approach to modulating the host immune response against biomaterials encapsulating pancreatic β-cells involves incorporating biological factors into biomaterial devices to reduce local inflammation and create immune-privileged sites [15, 17]. Immune-modulating molecules, such as cytokines, chemokines, or immune checkpoint inhibitors, can be incorporated into biomaterials to modulate the immune response

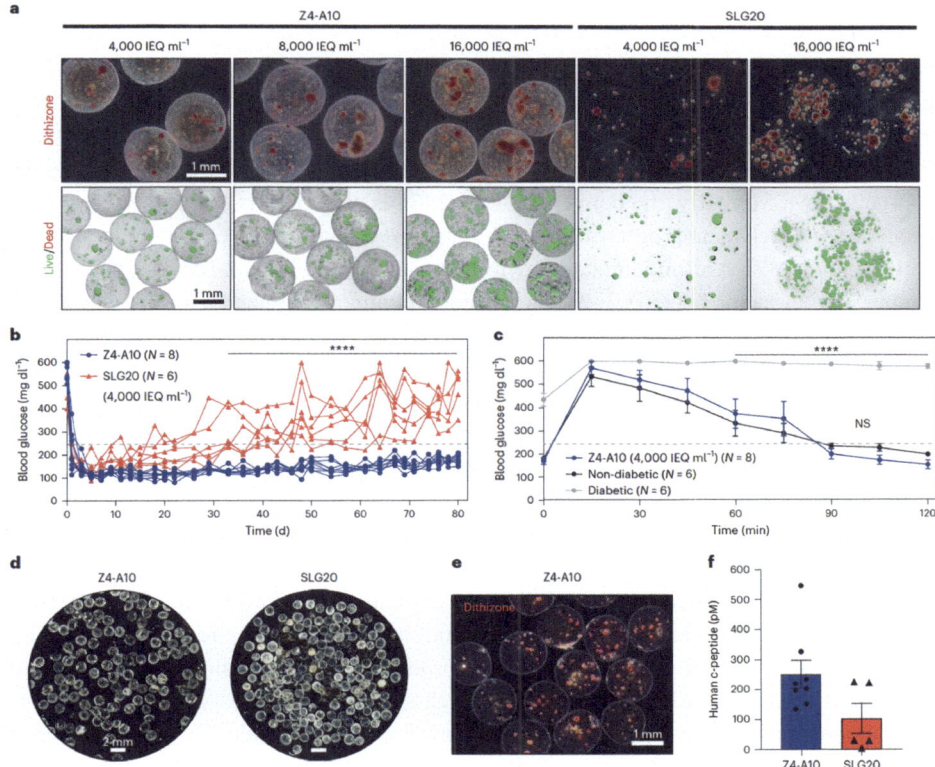

Fig. 3.4 Lead hydrogel encapsulating xenogeneic human islets demonstrates a diabetic reversal in immunocompetent C57BL/6 J mice. **a** Representative images of pre-implant capsules. Z4-A10 capsules containing human islets at a density of 10 IEQ per capsule, 20 IEQ per capsule and 40 IEQ per capsule, respectively. Z1-A34 and SLG20 capsules were used as control material. Dithizone staining indicates viable islets within the capsule matrix. After encapsulation, islets show good viability (live, green; dead, red). **b** Blood glucose levels for both Z4-A10 and SLG20 groups (4,000 IEQ ml − 1 density) were monitored until mice were euthanized (two-way ANOVA with Bonferroni multiple comparisons, ****P < 0.0001 (SLG20 vs Z4-A10)). **c** IVGTT test with Z4-A10 capsule (4,000 IEQ/ml) implant group in diabetic mouse, and non-implant group in diabetic mice and non-diabetic mice (two-way ANOVA with Bonferroni multiple comparisons; NS, not significant ****P < 0.0001 (all comparisons)). **d, e**, Representative dark-field (**d**) and dithizone staining (red, **e**) images of explanted Z4-A10 and SLG20 capsules (4,000 IEQ/ml). **f**, Human c-peptide measurements at 80 d post-transplantation (SLG20 vs Z4-A10). **Reproduced with permission** [7]. Copyright 2023, Springer Nature

to implanted materials. These molecules can be delivered locally to attenuate the local inflammatory response by polarizing macrophages toward an anti-inflammatory response or recruiting suppressive cell types [35]. For example, delivering CXCL12, an immunomodulatory chemokine, from alginate-encapsulated SC-β cells resulted in long-term insulin secretion without the need for immunosuppression [36]. CXCL12 acts by repelling effector T cells, recruiting regulatory T cells, and providing a pro-survival signal for β-cells [15]. Similarly, the delivery of CCL22 in islet allografts led to the recruitment of regulatory T cells and long-term protection against allograft rejection without affecting β-cell function [37]. Anti-inflammatory cytokines such as interleukin-10 (IL-10) and transforming growth factor-beta (TGF-β) can promote immune tolerance [38]. These cytokines can be delivered locally to the transplant site to reduce inflammation and promote tolerance. The localized delivery of TGF-β1 was shown to modulate the immune response to implanted materials and enhance cell function in T1D therapies [39]. Short-term release of TGF-β1 with islets reduced the infiltration of inflammatory immune cells and prolonged the survival of transplant islet allografts. In addition, soluble anti-inflammatory agents such as heparin [40], dexamethasone [41], and superoxide dismutase [42] can be incorporated onto biomaterials by surface coating, and these implant has shown the reduction of inflammation and fibrous encapsulation. Farah and Doloff et al. incorporated crystallized drug formulations within alginate capsules and showed suppressed FBR in rodents and non-human primates [6]. The authors investigated the effectiveness of utilizing crystallized drug formulations to mitigate fibrotic responses commonly associated with implantable devices. Traditional approaches, such as anti-inflammatory drugs or coatings, have demonstrated limited success in preventing fibrotic encapsulation. The researchers implanted devices coated with the crystallized drug formulation (GW2580, a colony stimulating factor 1 receptor inhibitor) and observed the animals over an extended period. The results indicated a significant reduction in fibrotic encapsulation around the implants, compared to the control group that received uncoated devices. Also, they examined how this combination affected xenogeneic islet transplantation. The alginate microcapsules containing GW2580 successfully released the immunomodulator over an extended period, leading to decreased fibrosis and improved regulation of blood sugar levels in mice that received islet transplantation (Fig. 3.5). However, the long-term effects and potential side effects of the crystallized drug formulations require careful evaluation. Further studies are needed to refine the formulation and dosage, optimize the release kinetics, and evaluate the long-term safety and efficacy in human subjects.

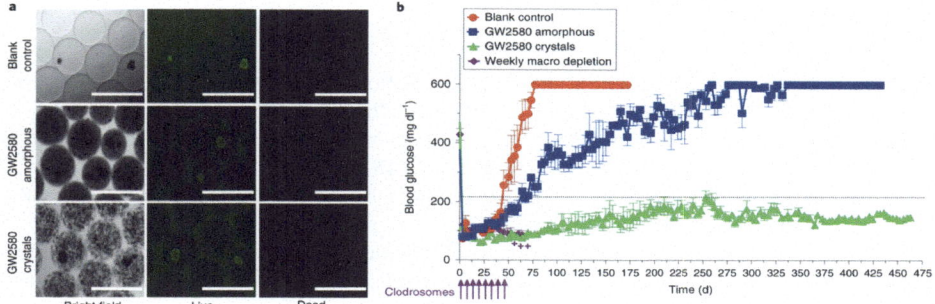

Fig. 3.5 Drug was co-encapsulated with islets (rat or human) and transplanted into STZ-C57BL/6 diabetic mice. **a** Live/dead staining confirming viability of rat islet cells with both amorphous and crystalline GW2580 prepared in ~500–600 μm alginate capsules. Scale bars, 1,000 μm. Image rows: same field of view, focus and magnification. **b** Blood glucose curves showing significantly prolonged normoglycemic maintenance with crystalline GW2580 (green), over blank (no drug, red) controls and amorphous-loaded (blue) capsules co-encapsulating 500 islet equivalents rat islets and transplanted IP. Macrophage-depleting clodrosomes (liposomal clodronate) were administered weekly (purple arrows) as positive control (++, group was terminated due to toxicity). Reproduced with permission[6]. Copyright 2019, Springer Nature

Table 3.1 Currently available diabetes treatments in T1D

Type	Function	Limitation
Insulin injections	• Most common treatment • Delay the onset/reduce the progression of diabetic complications	• Requires multiple daily injections, close monitoring, dose adjustment • Life-threatening complication (Hyperglycaemia/Hypoglycaemia)
Insulin pump	• Continued insulin treatment	• Requires constant patient attention • Cannot regulate blood glucose homeostasis
Pancreas transplantation	• Increasing success rate • Provide almost normal glucose homeostasis	• Requires life-long immunosuppressive medication • Donor shortage
Islet transplantation	• Restoring glycemic control • No major surgery required	• Needs chronic immunosuppression • Lack of cadaveric donor pancreas

References

1. Desai, T. & Shea, L. D. Advances in islet encapsulation technologies. *Nature Reviews Drug Discovery* **16**, 338-350, https://doi.org/10.1038/nrd.2016.232 (2017).
2. Ernst, A. U., Wang, L.-H. & Ma, M. Islet encapsulation. *Journal of Materials Chemistry B* **6**, 6705-6722, https://doi.org/10.1039/C8TB02020E (2018).
3. Association, A. D. Diagnosis and Classification of Diabetes Mellitus. *Diabetes Care* **37**, S81-S90, https://doi.org/10.2337/dc14-S081 (2013).
4. Li, Y. et al. In vitro platform establishes antigen-specific CD8+ T cell cytotoxicity to encapsulated cells via indirect antigen recognition. *Biomaterials* **256**, 120182, doi:https://doi.org/https://doi.org/10.1016/j.biomaterials.2020.120182 (2020).
5. J. Bauer, S. & Doloff, J. C. in *Immunomodulatory Biomaterials* (eds Stephen F. Badylak & Jennifer H. Elisseeff) 215–250 (Woodhead Publishing, 2021).
6. Farah, S. et al. Long-term implant fibrosis prevention in rodents and non-human primates using crystallized drug formulations. *Nature Materials* **18**, 892-904, https://doi.org/10.1038/s41563-019-0377-5 (2019).
7. Mukherjee, S. et al. Screening hydrogels for antifibrotic properties by implanting cellularly barcoded alginates in mice and a non-human primate. *Nature Biomedical Engineering*, https://doi.org/10.1038/s41551-023-01016-2 (2023).
8. Bochenek, M. A. et al. Alginate encapsulation as long-term immune protection of allogeneic pancreatic islet cells transplanted into the omental bursa of macaques. *Nature Biomedical Engineering* **2**, 810-821, https://doi.org/10.1038/s41551-018-0275-1 (2018).
9. Ernst, A. U. et al. Nanotechnology in cell replacement therapies for type 1 diabetes. *Advanced Drug Delivery Reviews* **139**, 116-138, https://doi.org/10.1016/j.addr.2019.01.013 (2019).
10. Hortelano, G. Therapeutic applications of cell microencapsulation. Foreword. *Adv Exp Med Biol* **670**, vii-viii (2010).
11. Ryan, A. J., O'Neill, H. S., Duffy, G. P. & O'Brien, F. J. Advances in polymeric islet cell encapsulation technologies to limit the foreign body response and provide immunoisolation. *Current Opinion in Pharmacology* **36**, 66-71, https://doi.org/10.1016/j.coph.2017.07.013 (2017).
12. Wang, X. et al. Local Immunomodulatory Strategies to Prevent Allo-Rejection in Transplantation of Insulin-Producing Cells. *Advanced Science* **8**, 2003708, https://doi.org/10.1002/advs.202003708 (2021).
13. Farina, M., Alexander, J. F., Thekkedath, U., Ferrari, M. & Grattoni, A. Cell encapsulation: Overcoming barriers in cell transplantation in diabetes and beyond. *Advanced Drug Delivery Reviews* **139**, 92-115, https://doi.org/10.1016/j.addr.2018.04.018 (2019).
14. Orive, G. et al. Engineering a Clinically Translatable Bioartificial Pancreas to Treat Type I Diabetes. *Trends in Biotechnology* **36**, 445-456, https://doi.org/10.1016/j.tibtech.2018.01.007 (2018).
15. Kim, B. et al. Current Advances in Immunomodulatory Biomaterials for Cell Therapy and Tissue Engineering. *Advanced Therapeutics* **n/a**, 2300002, https://doi.org/10.1002/adtp.202300002.
16. Paez-Mayorga, J. et al. Emerging strategies for beta cell transplantation to treat diabetes. *Trends in Pharmacological Sciences* **43**, 221-233, https://doi.org/10.1016/j.tips.2021.11.007 (2022).
17. Desai, T. & Shea, L. D. Advances in islet encapsulation technologies. *Nat Rev Drug Discov* **16**, 338-350, https://doi.org/10.1038/nrd.2016.232 (2017).
18. Steele, J. A. M., Hallé, J. P., Poncelet, D. & Neufeld, R. J. Therapeutic cell encapsulation techniques and applications in diabetes. *Advanced Drug Delivery Reviews* **67-68**, 74-83, https://doi.org/10.1016/j.addr.2013.09.015 (2014).

19. Desai, T. & Shea, L. D. Advances in islet encapsulation technologies. *Nature Reviews Drug Discovery* **16**, 338, https://doi.org/10.1038/nrd.2016.232 (2016).
20. Hwa, A. J. & Weir, G. C. Transplantation of Macroencapsulated Insulin-Producing Cells. *Current Diabetes Reports* **18**, 50, https://doi.org/10.1007/s11892-018-1028-y (2018).
21. Lim, F. & Sun, A. M. Microencapsulated islets as bioartificial endocrine pancreas. *Science* **210**, 908, https://doi.org/10.1126/science.6776628 (1980).
22. Dolgin, E. Encapsulate this. *Nature Medicine* **20**, 9-11, https://doi.org/10.1038/nm0114-9 (2014).
23. Jacobs-Tulleneers-Thevissen, D. *et al.* Sustained function of alginate-encapsulated human islet cell implants in the peritoneal cavity of mice leading to a pilot study in a type 1 diabetic patient. *Diabetologia* **56**, 1605-1614, https://doi.org/10.1007/s00125-013-2906-0 (2013)
24. Veiseh, O. & Vegas, A. J. Domesticating the foreign body response: Recent advances and applications. *Advanced Drug Delivery Reviews* **144**, 148-161, https://doi.org/10.1016/j.addr.2019.08.010 (2019).
25. Desai, T. A. & Tang, Q. Islet encapsulation therapy — racing towards the finish line? *Nature Reviews Endocrinology* **14**, 630-632, https://doi.org/10.1038/s41574-018-0100-7 (2018).
26. Lin, C. M. & Gill, R. G. Direct and indirect allograft recognition: pathways dictating graft rejection mechanisms. *Current Opinion in Organ Transplantation* **21**, 40-44, https://doi.org/10.1097/mot.0000000000000263 (2016).
27. Ali, J. M., Bolton, E. M., Bradley, J. A. & Pettigrew, G. J. Allorecognition Pathways in Transplant Rejection and Tolerance. *Transplantation* **96**, 681-688, https://doi.org/10.1097/TP.0b013e31829853ce (2013).
28. Hilburger, C. E., Rosenwasser, M. J. & Delcassian, D. The type 1 diabetes immune niche: Immunomodulatory biomaterial design considerations for beta cell transplant therapies. *Journal of Immunology and Regenerative Medicine* **17**, 100063, https://doi.org/10.1016/j.regen.2022.100063 (2022).
29. Stabler, C. L., Li, Y., Stewart, J. M. & Keselowsky, B. G. Engineering immunomodulatory biomaterials for type 1 diabetes. *Nature Reviews Materials* **4**, 429-450, https://doi.org/10.1038/s41578-019-0112-5 (2019).
30. Wang, X. *et al.* A nanofibrous encapsulation device for safe delivery of insulin-producing cells to treat type 1 diabetes. *Science Translational Medicine* **13**, eabb4601, https://doi.org/10.1126/scitranslmed.abb4601 (2021).
31. Liu, Q. *et al.* Zwitterionically modified alginates mitigate cellular overgrowth for cell encapsulation. *Nature Communications* **10**, 5262, https://doi.org/10.1038/s41467-019-13238-7 (2019).
32. Vegas, A. J. *et al.* Combinatorial hydrogel library enables identification of materials that mitigate the foreign body response in primates. *Nature Biotechnology* **34**, 345-352, https://doi.org/10.1038/nbt.3462 (2016).
33. Aghlara-Fotovat, S., Nash, A., Kim, B., Krencik, R. & Veiseh, O. Targeting the extracellular matrix for immunomodulation: applications in drug delivery and cell therapies. *Drug Delivery and Translational Research* **11**, 2394-2413, https://doi.org/10.1007/s13346-021-01018-0 (2021).
34. Vegas, A. J. *et al.* Long-term glycemic control using polymer-encapsulated human stem cell–derived beta cells in immune-competent mice. *Nature Medicine* **22**, 306-311, https://doi.org/10.1038/nm.4030 (2016).
35. Atri, C., Guerfali, F. Z. & Laouini, D. Role of Human Macrophage Polarization in Inflammation during Infectious Diseases. *International Journal of Molecular Sciences* **19**, 1801 (2018).
36. Chen, T. *et al.* Alginate Encapsulant Incorporating CXCL12 Supports Long-Term Allo- and Xenoislet Transplantation Without Systemic Immune Suppression. *American Journal of Transplantation* **15**, 618-627, https://doi.org/10.1111/ajt.13049 (2015).

37. Montane, J. *et al.* CCL22 Prevents Rejection of Mouse Islet Allografts and Induces Donor-Specific Tolerance. *Cell Transplantation* **24**, 2143-2154, https://doi.org/10.3727/096368914x685249 (2015).
38. Taylor, A., Verhagen, J., Blaser, K., Akdis, M. & Akdis, C. A. Mechanisms of immune suppression by interleukin-10 and transforming growth factor-β: the role of T regulatory cells. *Immunology* **117**, 433-442, https://doi.org/10.1111/j.1365-2567.2006.02321.x (2006).
39. Liu, J. M. H. *et al.* Transforming growth factor-beta 1 delivery from microporous scaffolds decreases inflammation post-implant and enhances function of transplanted islets. *Biomaterials* **80**, 11-19, https://doi.org/10.1016/j.biomaterials.2015.11.065 (2016).
40. Peng, Y., Tellier, L. E. & Temenoff, J. S. Heparin-based hydrogels with tunable sulfation & degradation for anti-inflammatory small molecule delivery. *Biomater Sci* **4**, 1371-1380, https://doi.org/10.1039/c6bm00455e (2016).
41. Zhong, Y. & Bellamkonda, R. V. Dexamethasone-coated neural probes elicit attenuated inflammatory response and neuronal loss compared to uncoated neural probes. *Brain Research* **1148**, 15-27, https://doi.org/10.1016/j.brainres.2007.02.024 (2007).
42. Udipi, K. *et al.* Modification of inflammatory response to implanted biomedical materials in vivo by surface bound superoxide dismutase mimics. *Journal of Biomedical Materials Research* **51**, 549-560, https://doi.org/10.1002/1097-4636(20000915)51:4<549::AID-JBM2>3.0.CO;2-Z (2000).

Cell-Based Therapies in Cancer 4

Andrea Hernandez and Sudip Mukherjee

4.1 Introduction

The immune system can respond to immunogenic pathogens and clear damaged cells. This constant surveillance offers protection to the human body from illnesses and infections. The immune system orchestrates which immune cells must be activated and when to arrive at the site of interest. The two arms of the immune system, the innate and the adaptive immune system, take this timing into consideration. The innate immune system is the first responder to the site of interest. Their primary function is to contain and eliminate pathogens locally. Additionally, innate immune cells such as macrophages and dendritic cells (DCs) collect antigens from pathogens and present them to the adaptive immune cells. This antigen presentation takes time for the immune system to develop antigen-specific cells to mount a robust immune response. While this may function in external invaders such as bacteria, fungi, and parasites as they have antigens dissimilar to the host, it becomes increasingly difficult with self-cells that no longer follow physiological functions.

Cancer cells are self-cells that grow uncontrollably without a signal from the immune system. If the growth is unchecked, abnormal cell accumulation can develop into tumors. Normal cells are responsive to the immune system and follow normal physiological

---

A. Hernandez
Katz Department of Oral and Maxillofacial Surgery, The University of Texas School of Dentistry at Houston, Houston, TX, USA

S. Mukherjee (✉)
School of Biomedical Engineering, Indian Institute of Technology (BHU), Varanasi 221005, UP, India
e-mail: sudip.bme@iitbhu.ac.in

© The Author(s), under exclusive license to Springer Nature Switzerland AG 2024
S. Mukherjee et al., *Immunomodulatory Biomaterials for Cell Therapy and Tissue Engineering*, Synthesis Lectures on Biomedical Engineering,
https://doi.org/10.1007/978-3-031-50844-8_4

processes such as programmed cell death through apoptosis. Apoptosis is essential in eliminating unwanted cells during development, aging, a homeostatic mechanism to maintain cells, and a defense mechanism when cells are damaged by pathogens or disease. Diseases such as cancer are notorious for evading apoptosis. Most cancer cells are derived from self-cells and express regular tissue markers, reducing the likelihood of mounting an immune response toward cancer cells.

With the complexity of cancer, different approaches are needed to treat patients. Most cancers, such as breast, kidney, and lung, can be surgically resected if they are easy to access, have clear surgical margins, and do not intervene with nonregenerative tissues such as cardiac muscle and the spinal cord. Patients with lung cancer have tumor resection and, within the first five years, can have recurrence from secondary primary tumors. Depending on whether the secondary primary tumors are genetically identical or dissimilar to the primary tumor results in a change of treatment. In head and neck cancer, 40% of patients with a primary tumor have a second one. Tumor heterogeneity makes it difficult to eradicate tumor growth as some clones from the tumor may be sensitive to intervention while others continue to grow.

Other standard-of-care modalities include chemotherapy and radiotherapy. A small proportion of the chemotherapeutic drugs delivered systemically reach the target site due to biological barriers. This route of administration will require frequent doses and increase the risk of toxic side effects. With limited exposure to the treatment, the tumor can develop resistance. As for radiotherapy, this modality relies on DNA-damaging radiation to eradicate cancer cells. Both treatment options can affect noncancer cells due to the nonspecific distribution of drugs or physical damage to surrounding healthy tissue. Additionally, many patients who undergo a combination of these treatments develop a weakened immune system, and it takes several months for the immune system to recover. Many survivors struggle with clearing bacterial or viral infections since they have a suppressed immune system. An ideal treatment would target cancer cells, restoring the immune system's capacity to recognize and reject cancer. Therefore, many researchers are now looking into immunotherapy strategies to target cancer.

4.2 Fundamentals of Cancer Immunology and Immunotherapy

Cancer Immunology

A significant part of cancer immunology is being able to distinguish when normal cells deviate from physiological processes. Typically, normal tissue cells conduct their specific function and expand to replace unwanted cells. In physiological conditions, normal cells stop growing when they sense other self-cells through contact inhibition. Meanwhile, contact inhibition is lost in cancer cells resulting in uncontrolled proliferation. These cancerous cells can invade and spread to distant sites resulting in metastasis. Cancerous cells adapt to stressful environments and use different nutrients than normal cells to survive. The cluster of these cells that form tumors requires a constant flow of nutrients and therefore secrete angiogenic signals to allow cancer to thrive. Understanding the mechanisms cancerous cells use to survive will enable the development of therapies with specificity.

Another aspect of cancer immunology is understanding the interactions between cancer cells and the immune system to develop innovative cancer immunotherapies. The tumors' composition can vary based on stage, cancer type, and individual. Therefore, understanding the specific tumor immune microenvironment (TIME) can provide insight into the treatment to administer. Some tumors with immune infiltration, hot tumors, are responsive to immunotherapy. While tumors with minimal immune infiltration, cold tumors, are difficult to target as immune cells are either not present, immune desert, or cannot infiltrate, immune excluded. The tumor cell's mutational burden can increase tumor antigenicity while enhancing evasion strategies to targeted treatments. Tumors hijack the immune system by sending signals to the immune cells that protect the tumor instead of attacking it. For instance, most cancer cells express programmed death-ligand 1 (PD-L1) to inhibit T cells. Tumors can also decrease major histocompatibility complex (MHC) class I expression to avoid being detected by cytotoxic T cells. Therefore, the specific tumor immune microenvironment characterization indicates which immunotherapy strategies will be more effective.

Cancer Immunotherapy

Cancer immunotherapy uses biological factors to elicit an immune response towards cancer cells. This type of treatment can mount a specific immune response to cancer without affecting the surrounding tissue, ultimately boosting immunological memory and reducing cancer recurrence. Immunotherapies like immune checkpoint inhibitors (ICI), oncolytic virus therapy, vaccines, and cell therapies are approaches to battling cancer. Cell-based therapies are rapidly advancing fields that transplant living cells that can secrete factors or directly interact with the tumor microenvironment to reverse the disease state. Researchers have used biological factors such as adoptive cell therapies, stem cells, and engineered cells to treat various cancers. Several publications have covered ICIs, oncolytic virus therapies, and vaccines and their impact on treating cancer [1–3]. In this book chapter, we will expand on current cell therapies and effective methods researchers use to deliver and sustain the release of living drugs (Fig. 4.1).

Adoptive cell therapies use immune cells to eliminate cancer. There are four different types of immune cell therapies: tumor-infiltrating lymphocyte (TIL) therapy, engineered T cell receptor (TCR) therapy, chimeric antigen receptor (CAR) T cell therapy, and natural killer (NK) cell therapy. In TIL therapy, tumors are surgically resected, then the lymphocytes are expanded *ex-vivo* to target the tumor specifically and finally reinfused back to the patient. The patient's T cells are depleted to introduce T cell therapy. To support

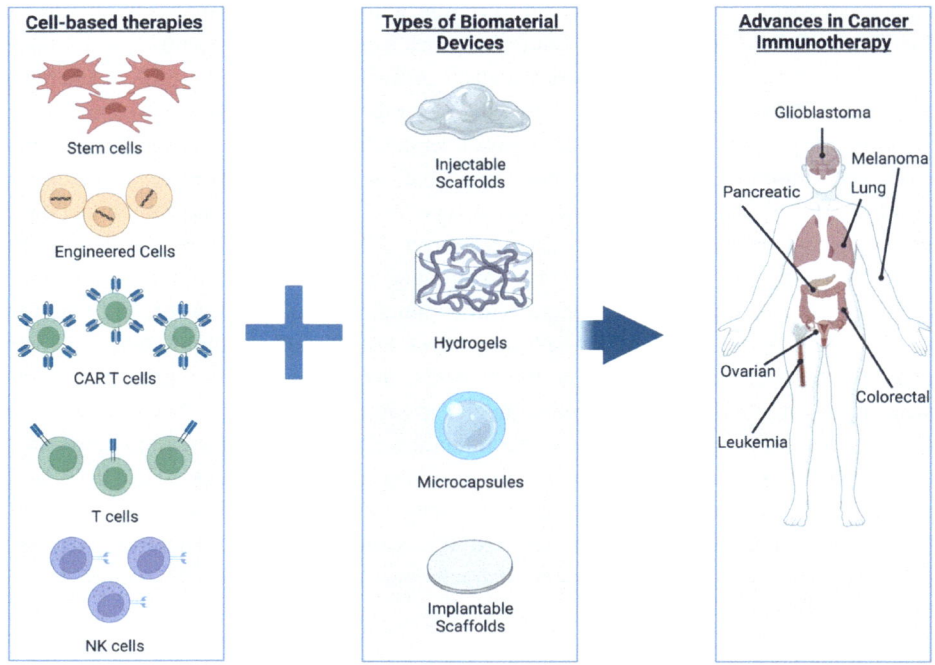

Fig. 4.1 Schematic illustration of biomaterial-assisted stem cells, engineered cells, CAR T cells, T cells, and NK cells for advances in cancer immunotherapy. Created in Biorender.com

the growth and activity of adoptive TIL transfers, infused TILs are combined with intravenous injection of interleukin-2 (IL-2). Since the treatment is personalized, wide-scale implementation is complex as it is labor-intensive and costly.

Immune cells can be genetically modified to target specific tumor markers. TCR, CAR T cells, and NK cells differ from TIL as the cell products can originate from patient-derived peripheral blood mononuclear cells and do not require IL-2 injections. The patient-derived peripheral blood mononuclear cells are easier to access than conducting tumor resections. TCR therapy can target tumor-specific antigens presented through MHC. Therefore, the patient's human leukocyte antigens (HLA) background must be considered for the TCR construct. The patients also undergo lymphodepletion and infusion of TCR therapy. CAR T cell contains an antigen-specific single-chain variable fragment from an antibody, a transmembrane domain, and an intracellular T cell signaling domain. CAR T cells do not require HLA matching like TCR therapy. NK cells can eliminate cells that lose MHC class I expression. Clinical trials have shown the overall safety of allogenic NK cell infusions, showing an opportunity to expand the use of NK cell therapies [4, 5].

Stem cells have self-renewing properties and can develop into many different cell types. Traditionally, stem cells have been used in tissue regeneration and are now applied to cancer applications [6]. Stem cells can migrate to micrometastatic lesions and be modified to express or release anticancer factors and therefore are of interest for cancer treatment [7]. For instance, human mesenchymal stem cells (hMSC) were cocultured with GBM cells, and the U87-MG cell changed phenotypic expression and saw a decrease in proliferation in the presence of hMSCs [8]. Additionally, cells can be engineered to express factors of interest. HMSCs were transduced with a recombinant adenoviral vector expressing the murine IL-12 forming MSC/IL-12 [9]. When MSC/IL-12 was systemically delivered, the human renal cancer cell line experienced reduced growth and significantly prolonged mouse survival. Before being applied clinically in cancer applications, the immunosuppressive qualities of stem cells that may facilitate tumor evasion from the immune system must be addressed [10–12].

Many of the currently used cell therapies have similar obstacles. A major challenge is that many cells must be generated for a relevant clinical dose. The large number of cells needed can result in toxic levels of systemic cytokine release and severe immune cell cross-activation. Cell-based therapies elicit an immune response when delivered systemically, especially if it is not HLA-matched for TCR cell therapies and is foreign to the site of interest [13, 14]. With many of these therapies, systemic delivery of cells can result in a lack of infiltration into the tumor. Therefore, delivery methods are required to control the release, protect the living drug, and localize the therapy.

Novel biomaterial approaches to cell-based therapies

Biomaterials are an appealing delivery method as they are biocompatible and can locally control the release of therapeutics. Researchers have applied biomaterial-based cell therapies in tissue engineering and successfully mediated local tissue regeneration and wound healing processes [15–17]. The primary goal of having these cells in biomaterials is to protect the cells from immediate immune rejection and use secreted factors or cells to modulate the environment for desired activity directly. Therefore, cell therapies in biomaterials are being actively used for cancer applications. Encapsulated cell therapies in biomaterials such as alginate, fibrin, chitosan, and hyaluronic acid (HA) will be discussed in the different types of cancers (Table 4.1).

4.3 Ovarian Cancers and Aplated Ovaries

Ovarian cancer originates in the reproductive tract, including the ovaries, fallopian tubes, and the peritoneum. There are several types of ovarian cancers, such as epithelial ovarian carcinomas, germ cell tumors, and stromal cell tumors. Epithelial ovarian carcinoma (OC) is the most common type of cancer and is typically diagnosed in advanced stages. Epithelial OC has a low response rate to immunotherapy due to its suppressive TIME and

Table 4.1 Overview of biomaterial-based cell therapy strategies

Cell-therapy strategy	Material type	Delivery method	Results and Applications	References
T cells expressing chimeric NK receptor for Rae-1	Alginate	Scaffold in the peritoneal cavity	Improved overall survival and proliferation of T cells	[18]
RPE cells expressing mIL2	Alginate	Capsules in the intraperitoneal space	Reduced tumor growth and prolonged survival	[19]
Granulosa and theca cells	Alginate	Constructs in omental pouches	Mimicked native ovarian structure and circulating hormones	[20]
B7-H3 CAR T cells	Fibrin	Gels in the intracranial resection cavity	Enhanced antitumor activity	[21]
hTERT-MSC	Alginate	Capsules medial to the tumor	Decreased tumor volume and percentage of vessel area in tumors	[22]
MSCs expressing TRAIL	Fibrin	Patches delivered in the resected cavity	Suppressed recurrence of GBM and improved the percent survival rates	[23]
T cell clone specific for gp100	Chitosan	Injectable CTGels	Eliminated the cancer cells in vitro	[24]
CAR T cells, IL-15 and platelets conjugated with anti-PD-L1	HA	Hydrogels in the resection cavity	Greater antitumor activity	[25]
CAR T cells and cdGMP	Alginate	Scaffolds in the peritoneal cavity	Higher overall survival	[26]
CAR NK cells expressing zEGFR	HA	Scaffolds implanted in the region of the resected tumor	Eradication of tumor and metastasis reduction	[27]

low mutational burden [28]. OC tends to metastasize in the peritoneal cavity and generate malignant ascites, which can ultimately affect surrounding abdominal organs [29, 30]. Current intervention for advanced OC, undergo debulking surgery in affected areas, such as internal reproductive organs. Upon resection, most patients undergo chemotherapy to reduce recurrence rates. Immunotherapy strategies should generate tumor-specific lymphocytes and reduce immunosuppressive cells, like myeloid-derived suppressive cells (MDSCs) or polarized M2 macrophages [31]. Encapsulated T cells and living cells engineered to secrete the therapeutic factor can be used to treat ovarian cancer.

T cells can be modified in the laboratory to target and eradicate the patient's cancer. T-cell therapies must be effectively delivered to the tumor to have antitumor activity. Matthias Stephan's group generated an alginate scaffold that provides and stimulates the adoptive T cells to the tumor site [18]. They found by using a stage 3 ovarian carcinoma, an ID8 tumor cell expressing VEGF, the scaffold-delivered T cells expressing chimeric natural-killer receptor specific for Rae-1, an antigen characterized by ID8-VEGF, had improved overall survival compared to intraperitoneal prestimulated T-cells. Additionally, the scaffold-delivered T cells increased more in the peritoneal cavity than the prestimulated cells after 12 days. Biomaterials should control release, locally deliver therapeutics, and sustain the therapeutic.

Engineering cells to express the therapeutic factor of interest can provide continuous delivery of the therapy. Nash et al. created a proinflammatory cytokine delivery system with engineered human retinal pigmented epithelial (RPE) cells to stably express mouse IL-2 (RPE-mIL2) and deliver in an alginate-based microcapsule [19]. These cells display contact inhibition and allow for a controlled dose of the therapeutic of interest. They could change the dose by the number of capsules they delivered. The efficacy of the encapsulated RPE-mIL2 was tested with the ovarian ID8-Fluc tumor-bearing mice, and mice treated with 100 and up to 200 capsules had more significant tumor regression than untreated mice (Fig. 4.2). RPE-mIL2 mice survived significantly longer than RPE, sham, and recombinant mIL2 treatment groups. The RPE-mIL2 treatment induces the expansion and proliferation of CD8 T cells. The findings resulted in a phase I human clinical trial in platinum-resistant ovarian cancer patients (NCT05538624).

Cell-based therapies can be used in artificial organ implants to increase ovarian function after cancer therapy or menopause. Loss of ovarian function can also result in a decline of oestrogen, a hormone the ovaries produce to maintain bone strength. This decrease can result in rapid bone loss and an increased risk of osteoporosis and fractures. Pharmacologic hormone replacement therapy (pHRT) consists of estrogen alone or estrogen and progestogen hormones treatment regimens. PHRT was discontinued as a treatment for ovarian function because of adverse effects such as breast and ovarian cancers. PHRT, when delivered at an ideal dose, frequency, and proper timing, had a beneficial impact, such as enhanced bone mineral density without the risk of developing cancer. Therefore, a therapy that can temporarily control hormones and restore the hypothalamic-pituitary-ovarian endocrine axis regulation system is needed. A cell-based hormone replacement therapy (cHRT) was created through alginate-based capsules that follow the native ovarian structure and circulating hormones [20]. This was accomplished by sequential encapsulation of the granulosa and theca cells in different biomaterial formulations. Granulosa and theca cells produce estradiol (E_2) and progesterone (P_4) in response to follicle-stimulating hormone (FSH) and luteinizing hormone (LH), which creates a feedback loop that controls the dose and time of circulating hormones. The ovariectomized (ovx) rats treated with the ovarian construct's plasma level hormones of E_2 and P_4 were significantly higher than untreated ovx rats. Both cHRT and ovary-intact rats had similar FSH and LH levels after

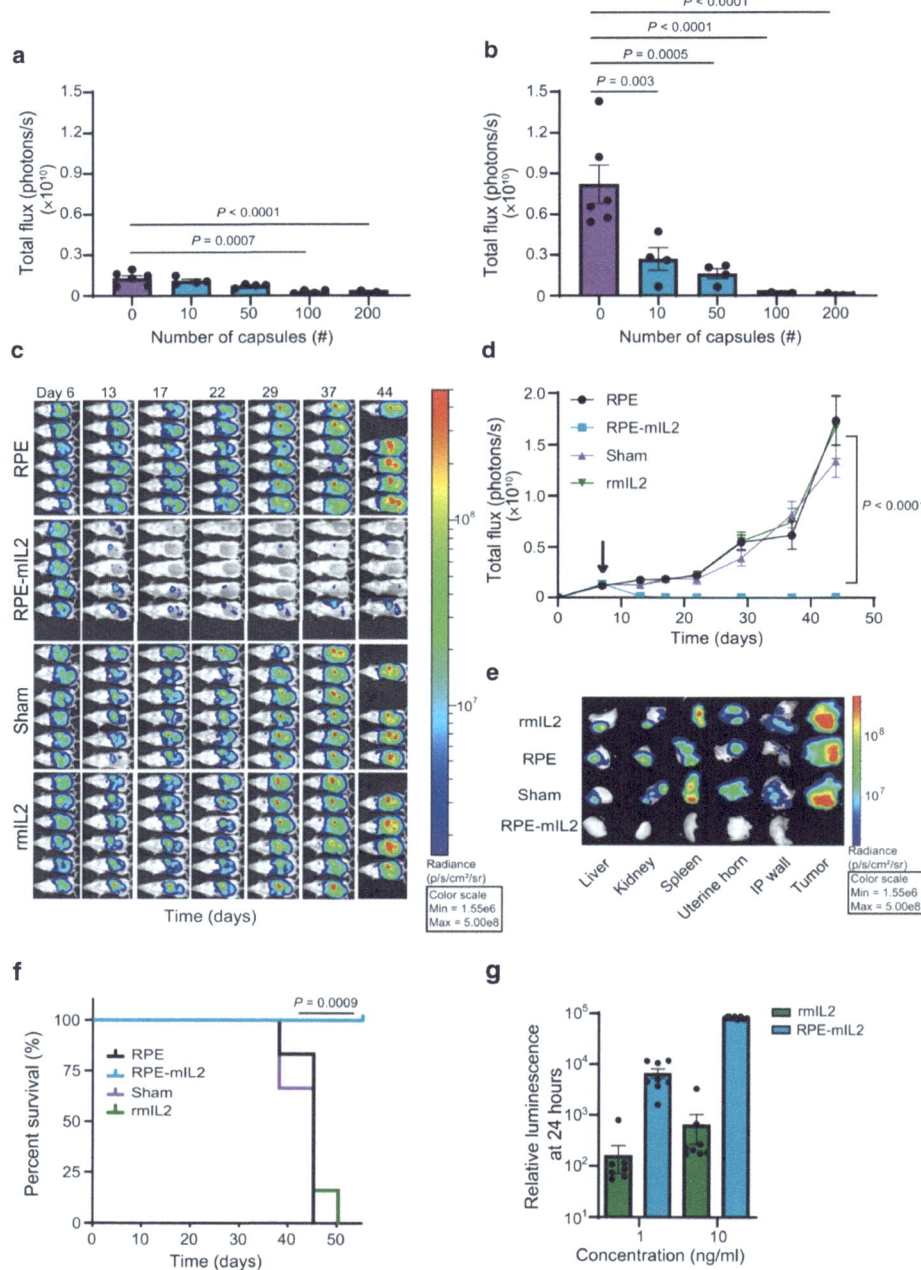

Fig. 4.2 RPE-mIL2 treatment has a significant effect in reducing tumor burden over time in ovarian cancer mouse models. Luminescent images tracking tumor burden as a function of RPE-mIL2 dose at **a** day 6 and **b** day 30 after treatment (means ± SEM). P values were determined using one-way analysis of variance (ANOVA) with the Holm-Sidak method for multiple comparisons. Data are from one dedicated experiment. **c** Luminescent images of mice (n = 5 to 6) over time. Data are representative of two independent experiments. **d** Tumor burden (n = 5 to 6) represented by total flux (photons/s) plotted over time. The black arrow indicates RPE-mIL2 administration (7 days after injection; means ± SEM). P values were determined by two-way ANOVA, using the Holm-Sidak method for multiple comparisons. **e** Explanted organs and tumors collected from the IP space. **c** and **e** were collected using an f-stop of 1.2, 15 s of exposure, and a field of view at 24 and 12, respectively. **f** Survival curves (n = 5 to 6) depicted as percent survival over time in days after tumor injection. Comparison of survival curves was done using the log-rank, Mantel-Cox test. **g** Relative luminescence of 1×10^4 isolated murine T cells 24 h (n = 8) after treatment with rmIL2 or mIL2 secreted from RPE-mIL2. P values were determined to be $P < 0.001$ using two-way ANOVA, using the Holm-Sidak method for multiple comparisons. Data are representative of two independent experiments. The figure and caption are reproduced after permission from Science Advances, 2022 [19]

3 weeks of treatment. cHRT led to better bone mineral density and bone porosity compared to pHRT. Encapsulating cell-based therapies can create organ constructs and deliver the necessary molecules to restore biological feedback mechanisms.

Glioblastomas

Glioblastoma (GBM) is an aggressive cancer that impacts brain tissue. The conventional treatment for GBM is tumor resection, radiotherapy, and chemotherapy with concurrent temozolomide [32]. GBM cells can infiltrate the adjacent normal brain tissues of the tumor, increasing the risk of tumor recurrence. Immunotherapy strategies such as CAR T cell therapy are being investigated in clinical trials for GBM but have limited detected CAR T cells in the tumor site (NCT02209376, NCT01454596, NCT01109095). CAR T cells have been infused intracavitary to overcome the blood–brain barrier and are given additional infusions in the ventricular system (NCT02208362). Stem cells, particularly MSCs, are also used in GBM. MSCs' innate tumor tropism, the release of immunomodulatory properties, and the ability to be genetically modified to deliver therapies are attractive characteristics for oncological use [33]. Loaded CAR T cells and stem cells in biomaterials are feasible ways to provide therapeutic factors to treat GBM.

Engineered CAR T cells can target GBM-specific antigens. A significant part of the ineffectiveness of current immunotherapy strategies is the lack of approaches to deliver and control the release of cell-based therapies locally [34]. CAR T cells were loaded in fibrin gels to release effector cells in the resection cavity [21]. The gel allows for the gradual CAR T cell release to ensure cancer eradication, and the fibrin gel's inherent wound healing properties can stimulate the repair of the cranial defect. In an intracranial GBM model using U-87 MG expressing GFP-firefly luciferase, the mice treated with fibrin gel loaded with B7-H3 CAR T cells improved antitumor effects of CAR T cell compared to intracavity B7-H3 antigen CAR T cell injection (Fig. 4.3). Additionally, T cell growth factors can be loaded onto the gel to sustain T cells and surpass immunosuppressive TIME. This method allows for the continual release of CAR T cells at the site of interest and encourages the regrowth of the resected cavity. Biomaterials, in this case, should incorporate activation and proliferation factors that can sustain the therapeutic to act on cancer and encourage the regrowth of normal tissue.

Encapsulation of modified MSCs has shown promise in reducing GBM. Glioma cells were co-transplanted with alginate-encapsulated MSC in immunocompetent rats to reduce tumor growth [22]. After tumor inoculation, rats were either administered empty alginate capsules, capsules-containing telomerase reverse transcriptase gene (hTERT) MSC without endostatin transfection, or capsules-containing endostatin producing hTERT-MSC (endoMSC). After 12 days, capsules-containing hTERT-MSC without endostatin transfection groups significantly decreased tumor volume compared to the empty capsules. Histology analysis showed that endoMSC significantly reduced the percentage of vessel area in tumors compared to capsules-containing hTERT MSC without endostatin transfection and empty capsules. GBM was reduced when MSCs and anti-tumorigenic peptides were encapsulated and delivered in vivo. The encapsulated MSCs used paracrine mechanisms to reduce GBM tumor growth, which may reduce targeted immune response compared to free MSCs.

The viability of MSCs releasing the cytotoxic agent TRAIL (hMSC-sTR) upon encapsulation of hMSC-sTR in fibrin patches delivered over tumor was compared to delivery in the resection cavity to decide which method would be practical to treat patients with GBM [23]. Quantitative bioluminescence imaging (BLI) in vivo showed that fibrin encapsulation had higher MSC retention than direct injection. MSCs directly injected had no detectable signal after 10 days compared to fibrin-encapsulated cells at day 28. After 1 week of having glioma cells transplanted into mice, the tumors were removed and were either delivered hMSC-sTR or hMSC-GFPRLuc in fibrin patches into the resection cavity. BLI showed GBM recurrence in hMSC-GFPRLuc fibrin patches compared to hMSC-sTR, which suppressed recurrence and improved the percent survival rates of rats. Using different delivery methods showed that hMSC-sTR encapsulated in fibrin is effective post-surgery in minimal GBM. Current cell-based strategies should consider their therapy's practicality and whether biomaterials can better facilitate this process.

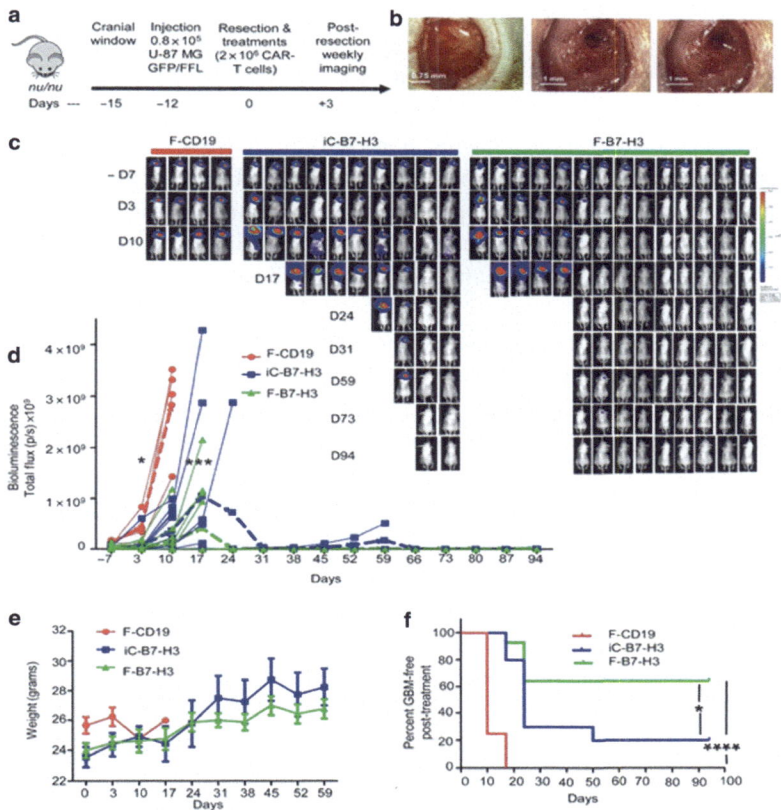

Fig. 4.3 CAR-T cells delivered via fibrin gel control GBM tumor growth after partial resection. **a** Schematic of the xenograft GBM model in which the tumor mass is partially resected and mice are treated with CAR-T cells inoculated via direct intracavity injection (iC-B7-H3) or by in situ formation of the fibrin gel (F-B7-H3). Control mice received CD19 CAR-T cells encapsulated in the fibrin gel (F-CD19). **b** Representative images showing tumor before resection (left panel), after surgery (middle panel), and after fibrin gel formed in situ in the tumor resection cavity (right panel). Scale bar, 0.75 mm - 1 mm. **c** Representative tumor BLI images showing tumor growth in F-CD19–, iC-B7-H3–, and F-B7-H3–treated mice. **d** Tumor BLI kinetics in F-CD19–, iC-B7-H3–, and F-B7-H3–treated mice (4 to 15 mice per group). *$P = 0.0296$ and 0.0471 for day −7 and day 3 versus day 17 in iC-B7-H3 versus F-B7-H3, (blue bold dotted line and green bold dotted line, indicating the averages respectively), determined by Turkey's multiple comparison test; ***$P = 0.0009$ as overall function calculated by two-way ANOVA. **e** Quantification of mouse weight in the experimental groups described in **b**. **f** Kaplan–Meier survival curve of the treated mice as described in **c**. *$P = 0.0259$ (iC-B7-H3 versus F-B7-H3); ****$P\ 0.0001$ (F-CD19 versus F-B7-H3), $\chi 2$ test. For the survival curve, mice were censored when the BLI signal reached 1×10^9 photons per second. Photo credit: E. A. Ogunnaike, University of North Carolina, Chapel Hill. The figure and caption are reproduced after permission from Science Advances, 2021 [21]

4.4 Colorectal Cancer

A complex network of cell types such as tumor-associated macrophages, MDSCs, CD8, and CD4 T cells infiltrates colorectal cancer (CRC). Tumor and stromal cells secrete chemoattractant, and the natural inflammation pathway draws these cells to the tumors. Cancer cells exploit stromal cells to promote tumor cell proliferation and metastasis. Ultimately the tumor has spatial and temporal control of the microenvironment that can be irreversible for stromal cells forming polyps along the wall lining of the colon. Over time, if the CRC enters the wall, it can infiltrate the lymph nodes or metastasize to other body parts.

Current immunotherapy treatments have applied cellular approaches such as NK cell and CAR T cell therapy to CRC [35]. A preclinical in vivo study found umbilical cord blood stem-cell derived NK cells (UCB-NK) had high antitumor cytotoxicity against RAS and BRAF mutant CRC [36]. Current limitations in treating metastatic CRC patients are related to resistance to anti-EGFR monoclonal antibodies; adoptive transfer of cytolytic UCB-NK cells can be a viable treatment option. An ongoing clinical trial provides intravenous CAR T cell injections towards CEA + CRC (NCT04348643). The extent of infiltration of adoptively transferred cells into the microenvironment of solid tumors, safety profile, and off-target effects against normal epithelial cells must be overcome to be widely used in the clinical setting.

The therapeutic index can be improved by providing a continuous supply of the interest factor. In addition to treating an ovarian tumor model, Nash et al. tested the efficacy of encapsulated RPE-mIL2 in MC38 tumor-bearing mice and found tumor regression after 1-week post-treatment [19]. To see if there was protection against tumor recurrence, they challenged the treated mice with a second MC38 tumor injection at a distant location (Fig. 4.4). They found that all treated mice did not develop a subcutaneous tumor and had a high percentage of CD4 memory T cells. Using this alginate-based biomaterial allows for the continuous production of IL-2 without additional administration and the gradual IL-2 termination by the natural foreign body response towards the implanted material. Additionally, they translated this cytokine factory to mesothelioma and found eradication of tumor burden in mice treated with a combination of RPE-mIL2 and anti-PD1 therapy [37]

4.5 Melanoma

Melanoma, like many other solid tumors, is heterogenous and resistant to conventional therapies. Targeted therapies such as BRAF and MEK inhibitors are used in melanoma to suppress tumor growth. The tumors can become resistant to targeted therapies and activate other survival pathways [38–40]. This is also the case in approved immune

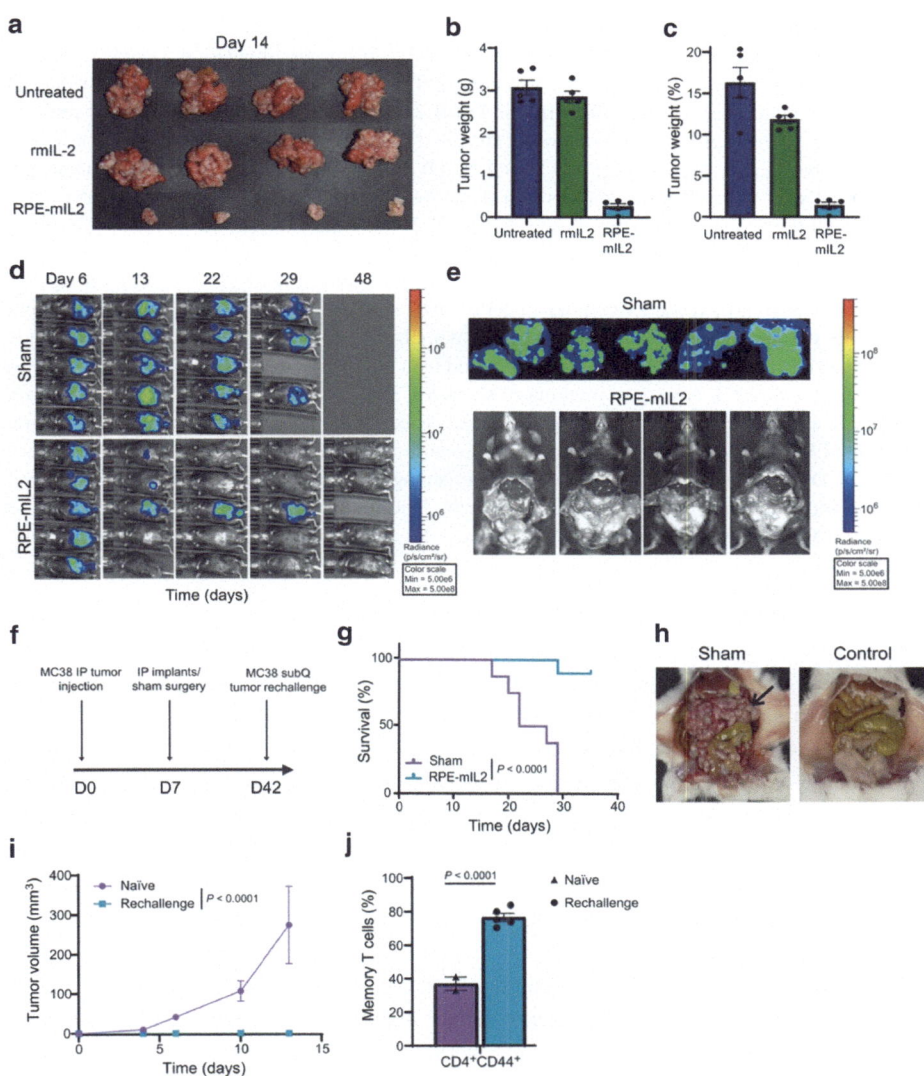

◄**Fig. 4.4** Cytokine secretion from RPE-mIL2 provides tumor reductive effects in an MC38 colorectal cancer model and protection from recurrence. **a** Visible IP tumors imaged at 7 days after treatment. Photo credit: Maria Ruocco, Rice University. **b** Tumor weights (means ± SEM). P values (P < 0.001 between untreated versus RPE-mIL2 and rmIL2 versus RPE-mIL2) determined by multiple comparisons test. Here, groups were randomly stratified before implantation. To account for heterogeneous variances, a Brown-Forsythe and Welch ANOVA test was used, with multiple comparisons using Dunnett's T3 test. **c** Tumor weights as a percentage of total body weight (means ± SEM). P values ($P < 0.001$ between untreated versus RPE-mIL2 and rmIL2 versus RPE-mIL2) calculated by one-way ANOVA, with Holm-Sidak's multiple comparisons test. **a** to **c** are representative of two individual experiments. **d** Luminescent images (n = 5) over time. I Ex vivo IVIS images of sham tumors (top) and exposed IP cavity of RPE-mIL2 mice (bottom) at day 57 after treatment. **d** and **e** From two independent experiments. **f** Schematic for subcutaneous (subQ) rechallenge study. **g** Percent survival over time. P value was determined by a comparison of survival curves by the log-rank (Mantel-Cox) test. **h** Necropsy imaging of sham MC38 mouse euthanized at humane end point versus naïve mouse. Photo credit: Michael Doerfert, Rice University. Black arrow indicates large tumor mass. **i** Subcutaneous tumor volume tracked over time. P value was calculated using one-way ANOVA. **j** CD3 + CD4 + CD44 memory T cell percentages. P values were determined by one-way ANOVA. **i** and **j** are from one dedicated experiment. The figure and caption are reproduced after permission from Science Advances, 2022 [19]

checkpoint inhibitors such as anti-CTLA-4 and anti-PD1 as the tumor immune microenvironment finds new resistance mechanisms [41, 42]. Some forms of resistance include impaired MHC class I antigen presentation, where adoptive cell therapies such as NK cells can eliminate dysfunctional cells [43, 44]. Cell-based therapies have advanced in melanoma clinical trials but have experienced delays due to toxicity. TCRs reacting to melanoma-associated antigens such as MART-1 or glycoprotein 100 (gp100) for metastatic melanoma were found to have responses ranging from 19 to 30% but also exhibited off-target toxicity in normal melanocytes (NCT00509288). CAR T cell specific for VEGFR-II observed severe adverse events in some treated patients (NCT01218867). Local delivery of cell therapies through biomaterials can eradicate these cancer types while minimizing the risk of toxicity.

Migration of TCR therapy from biomaterials and the ability of T cells to provide antitumor activity is necessary for further use in cancer treatment. An injectable chitosan-based biocompatible thermogels (CTGels) were generated at different concentrations of sodium hydrogel carbonate (SHC). They found the 0.075 M SHC (CTGel2) had the highest viability, proliferation, and escape compared to the other two SHC concentration CTGels [24]. In vitro CTGel-transwell recognition assay used a T cell clone specific to a melanoma antigen, gp100, presented by HLA-A2, encapsulated in CTGel2, and placed in the transwell above (Fig. 4.5). The CFSE-labeled melanoma cancer cells SK23-mel and 624-mel, both HLA-A2 + and gp100 + , were seeded below. Anti-gp100 T cells escaped the CTGel2, migrated to the bottom of the transwell, and executed their target cells, such as 624-mel and SK23-mel.

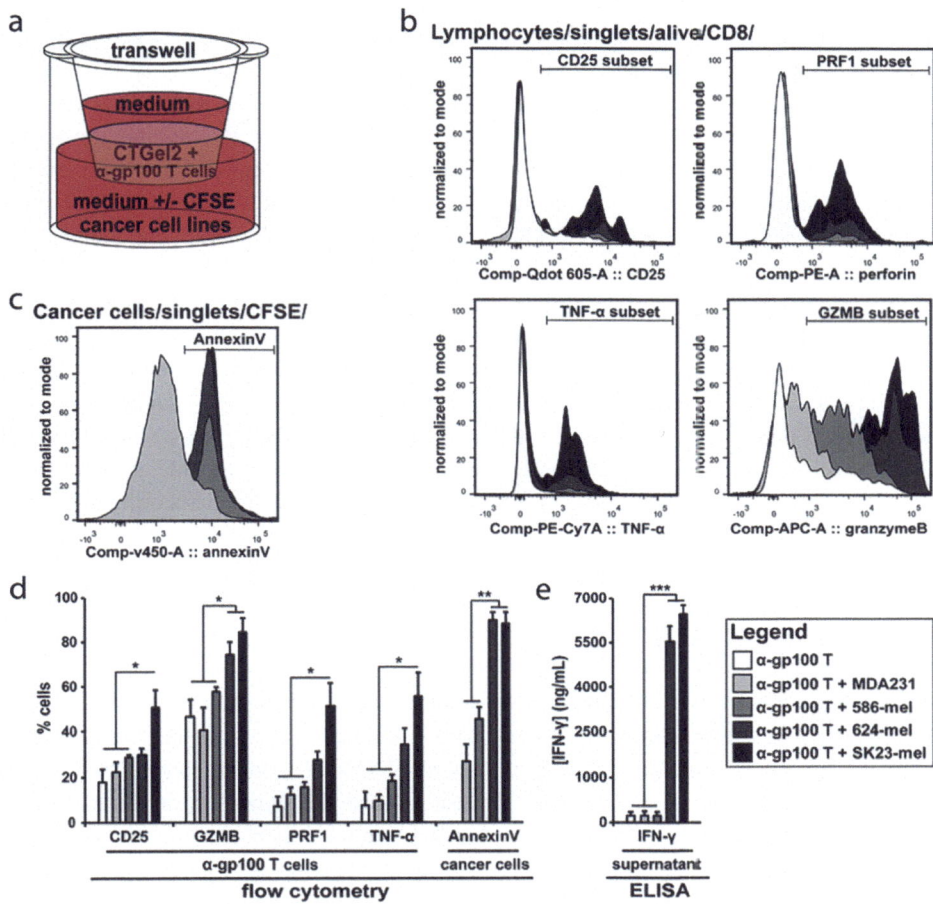

Fig. 4.5 CTGel2-transwell-mediated recognition/killing assay using α-gp100 T cell clone and melanoma cancer cell lines. **a** Depiction of transwell system illustrates how α-gp100 T cell clones were encapsulated in CTGel2 within transwells and CFSE labeled cancer cell lines were seeded at the bottom of the culture dish wells. Five days later, cells are collected from the medium at the bottoms of culture dish wells, and were split into two fractions for analysis. **b** Fraction one was analyzed using flow cytometry with gating strategy: lymphocytes (morphology)/singlets/alive/CD8, and then CD25, PRF1, TNF-α or GZMB. **c** Fraction two was analyzed using gating strategy: cancer cells (morphology)/singlets/CFSE + /AnnexinV. (**b–c**) FlowJo was used to generate normalized to mode displays of MFIs. **d** Percent cells expressing markers of interest are depicted in averaging graphs representative of two independent experiments preformed in triplicate. **e** Left, ELISA was used to assess the concentration of IFN-γ from the cell supernatants; right, legend provided for all figure panels. Bar graphs are representative of avg.±s.d. *$P < 0.05$, **$P < 0.01$, ***$P < 0.001$ determined by two-way ANOVA with Tukey's post-test. The figure and caption reproduced after permission from Biomaterials, 2016 [24]

Combinatorial strategies are necessary to treat complex cancers such as melanoma. A hyaluronic acid (HA) hydrogel reservoir that encapsulates CAR T cells targeting human chondroitin sulfate proteoglycan 4, highly expressed in human melanoma cells, cytokine IL-15 to maintain the activity of CAR T cells and human platelets conjugated with anti-PD-L1 was created [25]. After surgical resection of the tumor, the inflammation pathway would trigger the activation of platelets forming the platelet-derived microparticles (PMPs), releasing anti-PD-L1 and blocking PD-L1-expressing tumor cells. Concurrently, IL-15 facilitates the proliferation of CAR T cells and adoptive cell therapy-mediated activity. After the tumors were resected, the mice treated with the hydrogel containing CAR T cell, IL-15, and PMPs-anti-PD-L1 showed higher antitumor activity compared to the other treatment groups at 3 weeks post-inoculation in the resection cavity. Intratumoral delivery of CAR T cells is feasible in clinical settings but still struggles with T-cell distribution at the tumor site and can have side effects for antigens shared by non-cancerous tissue. Two different cell types were successfully loaded, indicating the ability to have different modes of cell-based antitumor activity. Using biomaterials that can include growth factors to maintain CAR T cells and additional immunotherapeutics will enhance the antitumor response.

4.6 Other Cancers

An essential consideration for cancer is ensuring tumor eradication and systemic antitumor immunity to prevent cancer recurrence. This could be done by incorporating adjuvant compounds, such as stimulator of interferon genes (STING) agonists, that stimulate antigen uptake and cross-priming of naïve T cells toward the tumor. In addition to their work in their ovarian model, Matthias Stephan's group used their alginate biomaterial to deliver tumor-targeting CAR T cells and provide a vaccine adjuvant, STING agonist cyclic di-GMP (cdGMP), in a pancreatic cancer model [26]. Scaffolds with cdGMP and tumor-specific CAR T cells had higher overall survival than scaffold-delivered cdGMP and control CAR T cells (Fig. 4.6). Many currently used immunostimulants require frequent administration and can lead to systemic toxicity. These biomaterials bypass injections by controlling the adjuvant's release over the tumor site.

Cancer treatments try to debulk as much of the tumor as possible, which can result in residual tumor left and reoccurrence. Therefore, additional immunotherapy strategies should be produced to eradicate the remaining cancer post-surgery. Several have looked towards NK cell immunotherapy as they can recognize the mismatch of inhibitory signaling pathways and can exert antitumor cell cytotoxicity [45, 46]. Some obstacles in NK cell therapy are the need to enrich cells and the higher targeting efficacy of tumors. A 3D-engineered hyaluronic acid-based niche for cell expansion (3D-EHANCE) was generated to treat leukemia [27]. Three different formulations of 3D-ENHANCE were tested to study the degradation and observe the morphological changes in cell culture conditions.

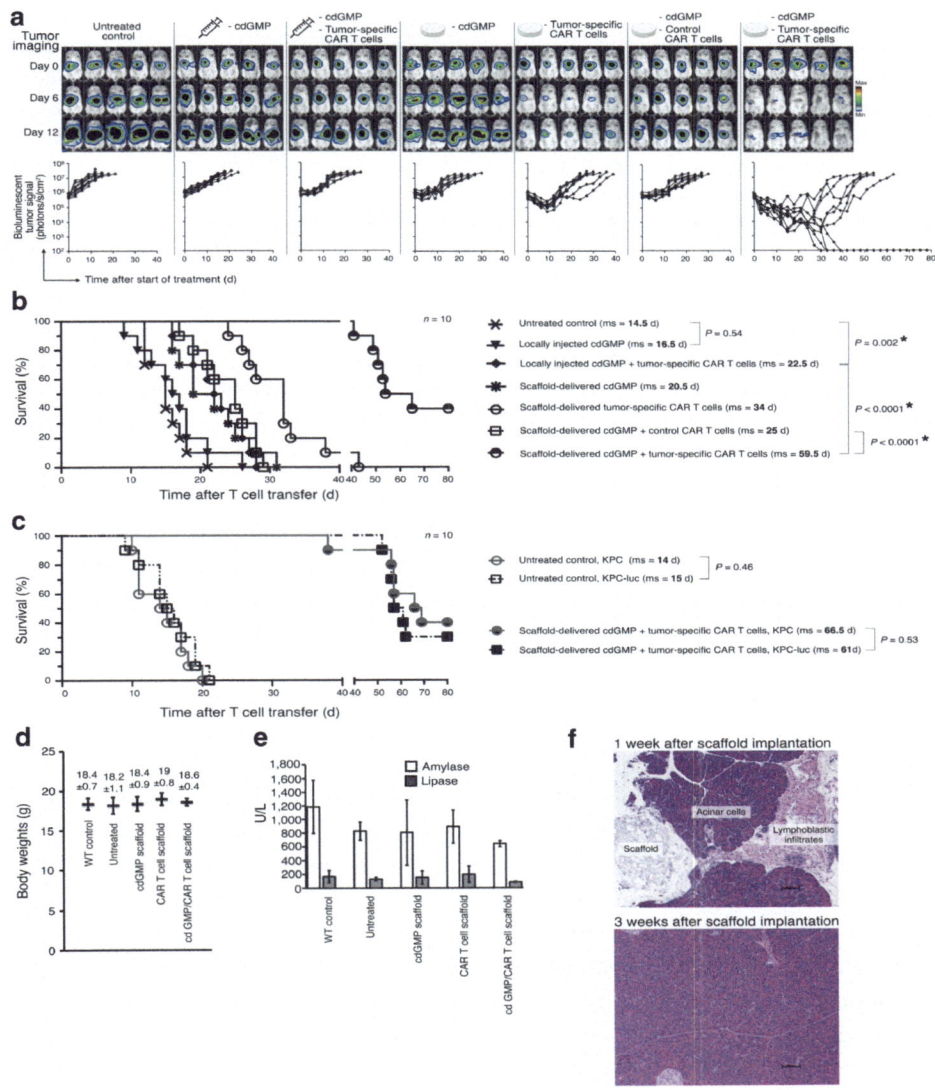

◀**Fig. 4.6** Implants that codeliver STING agonists along with CAR-expressing T cells can limit tumor immune escape in established inoperable tumors. **a** Serial in vivo bioluminescence imaging of KPC-luc tumors. Shown are 5 representative mice from each cohort ($n = 10$ mice in 3 independent experiments). Quantification of KPC bioluminescent tumor signals is also shown. **b** Kaplan–Meier survival curves for treated and control mice. Statistical analysis of the treated experimental and the untreated control groups was performed using the log-rank test, and a P value of less than 0.05 was considered significant. Asterisks indicate statistical significance. **c** Independent experiments showing survival and treatment responses of mice bearing unmodified versus luciferase-tagged KPC pancreatic tumors. Data obtained using the Log-rank test. **d–f** Assessment of side effects biomaterial implants have on pancreatic functions. **d** Average weight changes ($\pm$ SD) compared with control mice weights 1 week after treatment. Shown are 10 mice pooled from 2 independent experiments. **e** Serum levels of amylase and lipase. Each bar represents the mean $\pm$ SEM. **f** Representative H&E-stained sections of pancreas isolated from mice treated with the cdGMP/CAR T cell scaffold for 1 week or 3 weeks. Scale bars: 100 μm. The figure and caption reproduced after permission from The Journal of Clinical Investigation, 2017 [26]

3D-ENHANCE-2 degraded over 18 days and was used for the remainder of the study. From histological and mRNA expression, 3D-ENHANCE-2 contained zEGFR expressing CAR NK cells is necessary for tumor eradication and metastasis reduction (Fig. 4.7). These biomaterials can serve helpful in the prevention of solid cancers after resection.

4.7 Conclusions

Cellular therapies are an emerging treatment modality in cancer immunotherapy. The ability of cells to interact and adapt to physiological processes is an attractive option for the long-term administration of living drugs. These cells can respond to environmental stimuli and therefore modulate the amount of the therapy in the environment. CAR T, TIL, and NK cells are testing their efficacy in clinical trials. Local delivery and systemic toxicity are major barriers stemming from cell therapy clinical trials. To overcome this, some researchers have locally delivered cellular therapeutics to the tumor site but still require frequent administration for clinical responses. Biomaterials spanning from alginate, fibrin, chitosan, hyaluronic acid use a single administration of the cellular reservoir to treat cancer. The biomaterials can support both cell therapies and additional factors needed in maintaining the living drug in cases like the co-delivery of IL-2 with TIL therapy. Due to the loading capability of these biomaterials, the live therapeutics can be combined with additional immunotherapy strategies such as immune checkpoint blockade and other immunomodulators. Research should consider new ways to improve the delivery and regulation of therapies to have better clinical outcomes. Cell therapies in biomaterials hold promise in reducing systemic toxicity, providing a local and regulated supply of living drugs. Future research should consider new avenues of using long-term living medications in conjunction with biomaterial delivery methods to apply to other disease models such as diabetes and myocardial infarction.

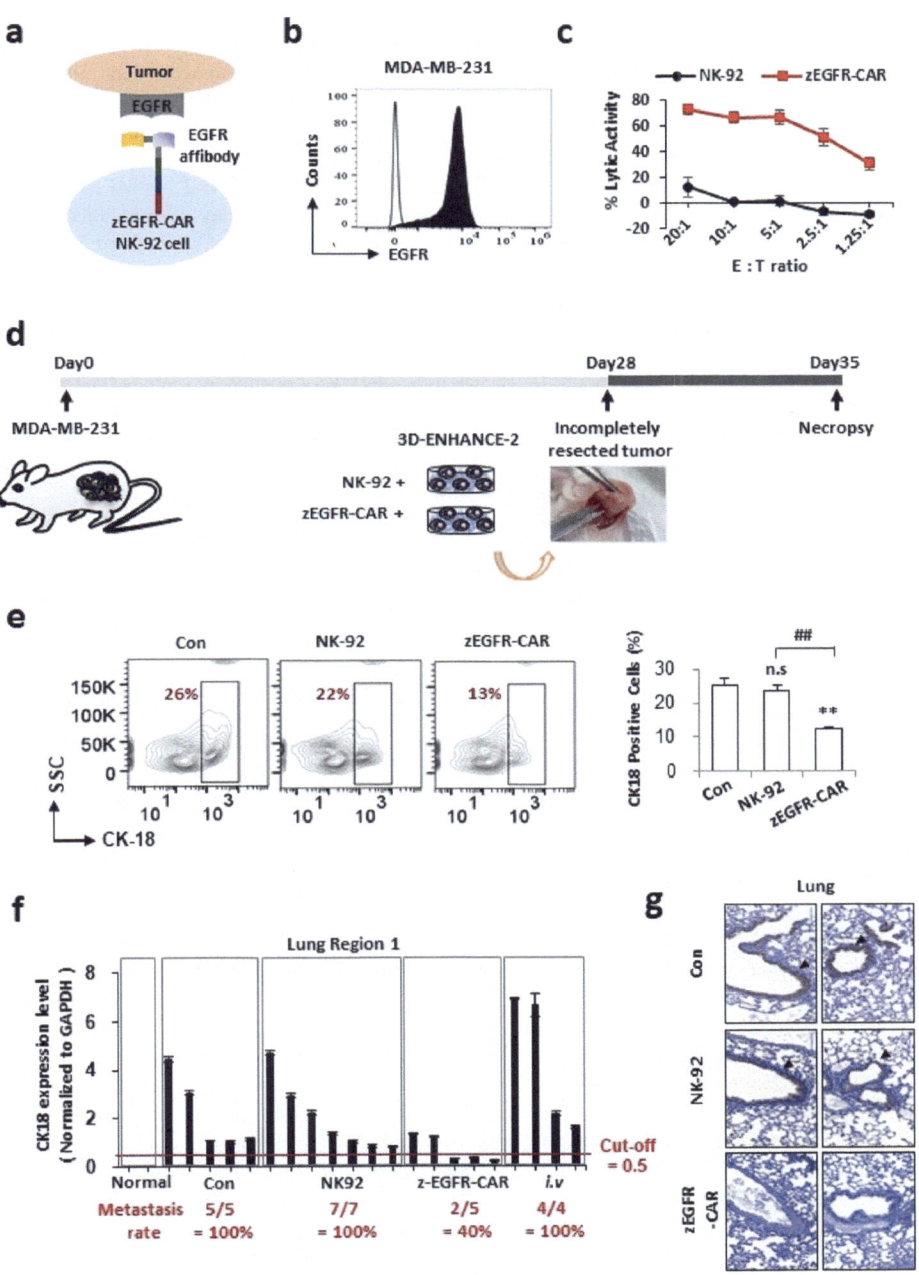

◀**Fig. 4.7** Perisurgical implantation effect of zEGFR-CAR NK cell-loaded 3D-ENHANCE on recurrence and metastasis of MDA-MB-231 xenograft. **a** Schematic of a zEGFR-CAR expressed at the NK cell surface. **b** EGFR expression levels of MDA-MB-231 tumors were determined using flow cytometry. **c** NK-92 and zEGFR-CAR cells were cultivated in 3D-ENHANCE-2 for 3 days, and MDA-MB-231 target cell killing was measured using Calcein AM-based cytotoxicity at different E:T ratios. **d** Experimental scheme. MDA-MB-231 tumors were orthotopically injected into the mammary fat pad of mice. DPBS (control group) and 3D-ENHANCE-2 cultivated with NK-92 and zEGFR-CAR NK were implanted at the tumor resected site at day 28 post-injection, and metastases were analyzed in lung tissues at day 35. **e** At necropsy, lung tissues from NK-92 and zEGFR-CAR NK-implanted mice (n = 3) were processed for flow cytometry using the gentleMACS tissue dissociation kit. **f** The percentage of mice bearing metastases in lung tissues are observed as the cutoff values based on the measurement of CK18 mRNA levels using qRT-PCR (n = 4–7). Additionally, zEGFR-CAR NK was intravenously injected in mice as a reference. **g** Immunohistochemistry stained with the antibody CK18. Brown indicates CK18 positive outcomes. The statistical significance differences of the data (*$P < 0.05$, **$P < 0.01$, ***$P < 0.001$) were determined against controls or $^{\#\#}P < 0.01$ against NK92 group (one-way analysis of variance). The data are representative of three independent experiment and expressed as mean ± SD (c) or mean ± SEM (e, f). The figure and caption reproduced after permission from Biomaterials, 2020 [27]

References

1. Liu, J., et al., *Cancer vaccines as promising immuno-therapeutics: platforms and current progress.* J Hematol Oncol, 2022. **15**(1): p. 28.
2. Rahman, M.M. and G. McFadden, *Oncolytic Viruses: Newest Frontier for Cancer Immunotherapy.* Cancers (Basel), 2021. **13**(21).
3. Robert, C., *A decade of immune-checkpoint inhibitors in cancer therapy.* Nat Commun, 2020. **11**(1): p. 3801.
4. Rubnitz, J.E., et al., *NKAML: a pilot study to determine the safety and feasibility of haploidentical natural killer cell transplantation in childhood acute myeloid leukemia.* J Clin Oncol, 2010. **28**(6): p. 955-9.
5. Sakamoto, N., et al., *Phase I clinical trial of autologous NK cell therapy using novel expansion method in patients with advanced digestive cancer.* J Transl Med, 2015. **13**: p. 277.
6. Chu, D.T., et al., *Recent Progress of Stem Cell Therapy in Cancer Treatment: Molecular Mechanisms and Potential Applications.* Cells, 2020. **9**(3).
7. Stuckey, D.W. and K. Shah, *Stem cell-based therapies for cancer treatment: separating hope from hype.* Nat Rev Cancer, 2014. **14**(10): p. 683-91.
8. Motaln, H., et al., *Human mesenchymal stem cells exploit the immune response mediating chemokines to impact the phenotype of glioblastoma.* Cell Transplant, 2012. **21**(7): p. 1529-45.
9. Gao, P., et al., *Therapeutic potential of human mesenchymal stem cells producing IL-12 in a mouse xenograft model of renal cell carcinoma.* Cancer Lett, 2010. **290**(2): p. 157-66.
10. Bajetto, A., et al., *Cross talk between mesenchymal and glioblastoma stem cells: Communication beyond controversies.* Stem Cells Transl Med, 2020. **9**(11): p. 1310-1330.
11. Mohr, A. and R. Zwacka, *The future of mesenchymal stem cell-based therapeutic approaches for cancer - From cells to ghosts.* Cancer Lett, 2018. **414**: p. 239-249.
12. Momin, E.N., et al., *The Oncogenic Potential of Mesenchymal Stem Cells in the Treatment of Cancer: Directions for Future Research.* Curr Immunol Rev, 2010. **6**(2): p. 137-148.

13. Betof-Warner, A., R.J. Sullivan, and A. Sarnaik, *Adoptive Cell Transfer and Vaccines in Melanoma: The Horizon Comes Into View.* Am Soc Clin Oncol Educ Book, 2022. **42**: p. 1-8.
14. Mo, F., et al., *Taking T-Cell Oncotherapy Off-the-Shelf.* Trends Immunol, 2021. **42**(3): p. 261-272.
15. Dolatshahi-Pirouz, A., et al., *A combinatorial cell-laden gel microarray for inducing osteogenic differentiation of human mesenchymal stem cells.* Sci Rep, 2014. **4**: p. 3896.
16. Facklam, A.L., L.R. Volpatti, and D.G. Anderson, *Biomaterials for Personalized Cell Therapy.* Adv Mater, 2020. **32**(13): p. e1902005.
17. Sharif, S., et al., *Collagen-coated nano-electrospun PCL seeded with human endometrial stem cells for skin tissue engineering applications.* J Biomed Mater Res B Appl Biomater, 2018. **106**(4): p. 1578-1586.
18. Stephan, S.B., et al., *Biopolymer implants enhance the efficacy of adoptive T-cell therapy.* Nat Biotechnol, 2015. **33**(1): p. 97-101.
19. Nash, A.M., et al., *Clinically translatable cytokine delivery platform for eradication of intraperitoneal tumors.* Sci Adv, 2022. **8**(9): p. eabm1032.
20. Sittadjody, S., et al., *In vivo transplantation of 3D encapsulated ovarian constructs in rats corrects abnormalities of ovarian failure.* Nat Commun, 2017. **8**(1): p. 1858.
21. Ogunnaike, E.A., et al., *Fibrin gel enhances the antitumor effects of chimeric antigen receptor T cells in glioblastoma.* Sci Adv, 2021. **7**(41): p. eabg5841.
22. Kleinschmidt, K., et al., *Alginate encapsulated human mesenchymal stem cells suppress syngeneic glioma growth in the immunocompetent rat.* J Microencapsul, 2011. **28**(7): p. 621-7.
23. Bago, J.R., et al., *Fibrin matrices enhance the transplant and efficacy of cytotoxic stem cell therapy for post-surgical cancer.* Biomaterials, 2016. **84**: p. 42-53.
24. Monette, A., et al., *Chitosan thermogels for local expansion and delivery of tumor-specific T lymphocytes towards enhanced cancer immunotherapies.* Biomaterials, 2016. **75**: p. 237-249.
25. Hu, Q., et al., *Inhibition of post-surgery tumour recurrence via a hydrogel releasing CAR-T cells and anti-PDL1-conjugated platelets.* Nat Biomed Eng, 2021. **5**(9): p. 1038-1047.
26. Smith, T.T., et al., *Biopolymers codelivering engineered T cells and STING agonists can eliminate heterogeneous tumors.* J Clin Invest, 2017. **127**(6): p. 2176-2191.
27. Ahn, Y.H., et al., *A three-dimensional hyaluronic acid-based niche enhances the therapeutic efficacy of human natural killer cell-based cancer immunotherapy.* Biomaterials, 2020. **247**: p. 119960.
28. Shen, J., et al., *Comprehensive Landscape of Ovarian Cancer Immune Microenvironment Based on Integrated Multi-Omics Analysis.* Front Oncol, 2021. **11**: p. 685065.
29. Macpherson, A.M., et al., *Epithelial Ovarian Cancer and the Immune System: Biology, Interactions, Challenges and Potential Advances for Immunotherapy.* J Clin Med, 2020. **9**(9).
30. Ning, F., C.B. Cole, and C.M. Annunziata, *Driving Immune Responses in the Ovarian Tumor Microenvironment.* Front Oncol, 2020. **10**: p. 604084.
31. Zhang, X.W., et al., *CAR-T Cells in the Treatment of Ovarian Cancer: A Promising Cell Therapy.* Biomolecules, 2023. **13**(3).
32. Bahadur, S., et al., *Current promising treatment strategy for glioblastoma multiform: A review.* Oncol Rev, 2019. **13**(2): p. 417.
33. Lin, W., et al., *Mesenchymal Stem Cells and Cancer: Clinical Challenges and Opportunities.* Biomed Res Int, 2019. **2019**: p. 2820853.
34. Abadi, B., et al., *Smart biomaterials to enhance the efficiency of immunotherapy in glioblastoma: State of the art and future perspectives.* Adv Drug Deliv Rev, 2021. **179**: p. 114035.
35. Ganesh, K., et al., *Immunotherapy in colorectal cancer: rationale, challenges and potential.* Nat Rev Gastroenterol Hepatol, 2019. **16**(6): p. 361-375.

36. Veluchamy, J.P., et al., *In Vivo Efficacy of Umbilical Cord Blood Stem Cell-Derived NK Cells in the Treatment of Metastatic Colorectal Cancer.* Front Immunol, 2017. **8**: p. 87.
37. Nash, A.M., et al., *Activation of Adaptive and Innate Immune Cells via Localized IL2 Cytokine Factories Eradicates Mesothelioma Tumors.* Clin Cancer Res, 2022. **28**(23): p. 5121-5135.
38. Konieczkowski, D.J., et al., *A melanoma cell state distinction influences sensitivity to MAPK pathway inhibitors.* Cancer Discov, 2014. **4**(7): p. 816-27.
39. Liu, X., et al., *KDM5B Promotes Drug Resistance by Regulating Melanoma-Propagating Cell Subpopulations.* Mol Cancer Ther, 2019. **18**(3): p. 706-717.
40. Manzano, J.L., et al., *Resistant mechanisms to BRAF inhibitors in melanoma.* Ann Transl Med, 2016. **4**(12): p. 237.
41. Machiraju, D., S. Schafer, and J.C. Hassel, *Potential Reasons for Unresponsiveness to Anti-PD1 Immunotherapy in Young Patients with Advanced Melanoma.* Life (Basel), 2021. **11**(12).
42. Thornton, J., et al., *Mechanisms of Immunotherapy Resistance in Cutaneous Melanoma: Recognizing a Shapeshifter.* Front Oncol, 2022. **12**: p. 880876.
43. Chang, Z.L., et al., *Rewiring T-cell responses to soluble factors with chimeric antigen receptors.* Nat Chem Biol, 2018. **14**(3): p. 317-324.
44. Lim, S.Y., et al., *The molecular and functional landscape of resistance to immune checkpoint blockade in melanoma.* Nat Commun, 2023. **14**(1): p. 1516.
45. Chiossone, L., et al., *Natural killer cells and other innate lymphoid cells in cancer.* Nat Rev Immunol, 2018. **18**(11): p. 671-688.
46. O'Brien, K.L. and D.K. Finlay, *Immunometabolism and natural killer cell responses.* Nat Rev Immunol, 2019. **19**(5): p. 282-290.

Cell-Based Therapies in Myocardial Infarction and Tissue Regeneration

Andrea Hernandez and Sudip Mukherjee

5.1 Introduction

There has been a surge of attention in cell-based therapies due to their ability to continuously supply healing agents, compatibility with the co-delivery of growth factors, and the capability to engineer cells to express the characteristic of interest. Some cellular therapeutics applied to cardiology, diabetes, musculoskeletal and spinal injury are mesenchymal stem cells (MSCs), beta cells, Schwann cells, and lymphocytes [1–4]. In myocardial infarction (MI) and tissue regeneration applications, stem cells and cells engineered to secrete growth factors are explored.

The post-myocardial infarction and tissue regeneration fields need treatment modalities that incorporates the regeneration process. After a MI, the injured mature heart cannot compensate for the loss of cells such as cardiomyocytes (CM) [5, 6]. Currently, heart attack survivors are given clot dissolving drugs, painkillers and antihypertensive drugs to lower the risk of a second event, but does not address the damage of the heart. Cell-based therapy is an attractive option to replenish the lost cells and restore the function of the damaged myocardium. The regeneration of the myocardium can be influenced by cells in a paracrine manner resulting in an improved ventricular ejection function and increased vascularization. When permanent tissues are heavily injured, they are removed and replaced

A. Hernandez
Katz Department of Oral and Maxillofacial Surgery, The University of Texas School of Dentistry at Houston, Houston, TX, USA

S. Mukherjee (✉)
School of Biomedical Engineering, Indian Institute of Technology (BHU), Varanasi 221005, UP, India
e-mail: sudip.bme@iitbhu.ac.in

with an organ transplant. Unfortunately, finding a match for a whole organ transplant and the successes with artificial implants are limited. Thus, biological substitutes, notably cells, are being investigated to restore tissue and organ damage.

Cells are mendable living drugs that can be engineered to express the therapeutic factor of interest and tailor the immune response. Some growth factors, such as vascular endothelial growth factor (VEGF), are therapeutic factors that can stimulate cell proliferation, wound healing, and angiogenesis. The living drugs must be sustained, which may require additional growth factors to thrive in the disease-state environment. Cells can be co-delivered with growth factors to reap benefits for succeeding in the environment and recruiting different cells to aid in the regeneration process. The activation of several regenerative pathways can result in tissue restoration.

Several challenges arise when administering cell-based therapies and should be addressed before widespread clinical translation. Typically, when cells and additional growth factors are allocated to the site of interest, the immune system can mount an immune response towards the therapeutic terminating the treatment, resulting in severe side effects. For example, a bacterial cell-based therapeutic could enter the epithelium and cause infection if not locally contained to the site of interest [7]. Unfortunately, clinical cell transplants are ineffective because they cannot be retained and protected. The cell's differentiation cannot be controlled due to shear stress during injection and exposure to the disease-state environment. Researchers are overcoming these obstacles by delivering cell-based therapies in biomaterials to protect them from the immune system and ensure the delivery of therapeutic factors. In this book chapter, we will discuss current cell therapies and biomaterial approaches to deliver and control the release of living drugs (Fig. 5.1).

Biomaterials are applied to cell therapies in tissue engineering as they provide a scaffold for tissue regeneration and can locally release wound healing factors. In post-MI and tissue regeneration, biomaterials are inherently practical for maintaining the structure of different tissue types. Additionally, biomaterials are used to mitigate the loss of injected cells to enhance cell–cell and cell-material interaction. Natural materials are typically biodegradable, so there must be a balance of adhesion of cells to the biomaterial and rate of degradation to promote new tissue formation [8–10]. For example, a self-assembling peptide, SLac, was used for functional tissue replacement and spatiotemporally directed differentiation for mouse embryonic stem cells [11]. The mouse embryonic stem cells had high viability, proliferation, and the cluster size significantly increased at each time point within the SLac. Furthermore, mouse embryonic stem cells differentiated into all 3 germ layers, indicating self-assembling peptide hydrogel can be used as a pluripotent stem cell differentiation platform. The self-assembling peptide hydrogel illustrated that it was biocompatible with pluripotent stem cells and fostered cell survival, attachment, and proliferation for up to 4 weeks. Many types of biomaterials carry cells, such as patches, capsules, and hydrogels. This book chapter will discuss cells loaded with materials such as alginate, fibrin, polyethylene glycol (PEG), chitosan, collagen, hyaluronic acid (HA),

5 Cell-Based Therapies in Myocardial Infarction and Tissue Regeneration

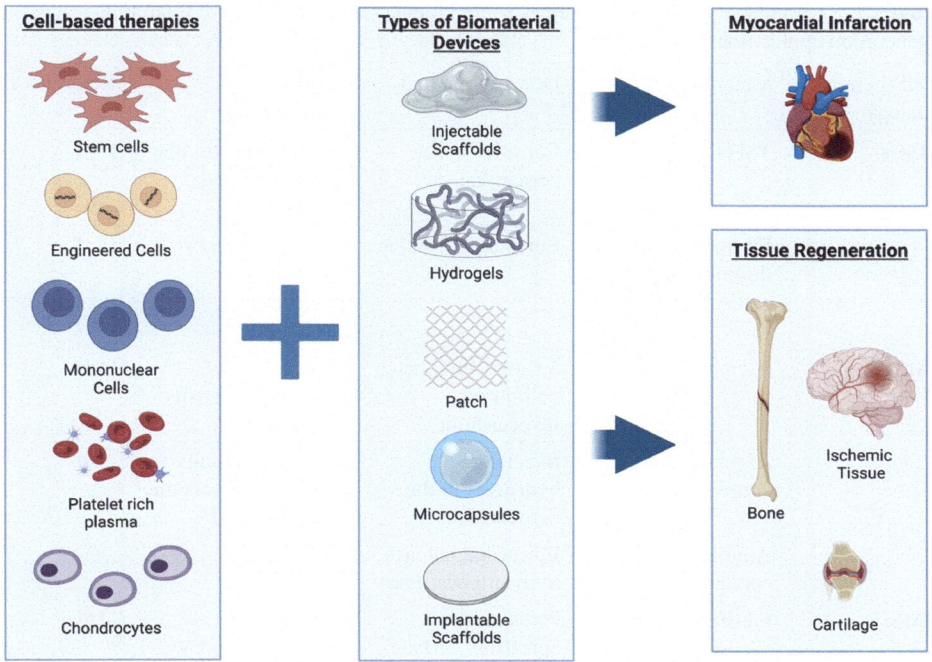

Fig. 5.1 Schematic illustration of biomaterial-assisted stem cells, engineered cells, mononuclear cells, platelet-rich plasma, and chondrocytes for applications in myocardial infarction and tissue regeneration. Created in Biorender.com

P-11$_4$, and peptide amphiphiles (PA) in tissue regeneration and myocardial infarction applications (Table 5.1).

5.2 Cell-Based Therapies in Myocardial Infarction

Myocardial infarction appears when a portion of the myocardium has a decrease in blood flow. Plaques and inflammation can restrict major blood vessels from sending blood, oxygen, and nutrients to the heart. As the arteries build up with plaque, less blood is transported to the heart, resulting in blocked arteries and, in extreme cases, a myocardial infarction. The current treatments for MI are aspirin, injection of clot-dissolving drugs, painkillers, and antihypertensive drugs to lower blood pressure and improve oxygen levels [26–28]. Extensive myocardial remodeling changes the heart's size, shape, and function upon cardiac injury. Ultimately, these changes can result in ventricular dysfunction [29, 30]. Hence, preservation and restoration of ventricular function are necessary. Cell-based

Table 5.1 Overview of cell-based therapies using biomaterials in myocardial infarction and tissue regeneration applications

Cell-therapy strategy	Material type	Delivery method	Results and Applications	References
MSCs	TMTD alginate	Capsules in the pericardial sac	Improved ventricular functioning and remodeling	[12]
	Fibrinogen and thrombin with collagen-sheets	Epicardial dressing	Reduced infarct size and increased neo-vascular formation	[13]
hMSCs	Alginate	Secured PEG patch on injured myocardium	Amplified total microvessel density	[14]
	Alginate and chitosan/B-GP	Injectable hydrogels in the myocardium	Increased viability in hypoxic and ischemic conditions and retained cells	[15]
	Alginate and collagen	Epicardial patches in the myocardium		
BMSCs	Fibrin	Patch on the epicardial surface	Enhanced post-infarction LV function	[16]
hiPSCs	Fibrin	Cardiac muscle patch	Improved in LVF, infarct size, and myocardial wall stress	[17]
CHO secrete VEGF	APA	Capsules in intramyocardial injection around the infarcted region	Declined fractional shortening and LV enlargement	[18]
HBMSC	Alginate-$VEGF_{165}$/ PDLLA-BMP-2	Scaffolds in femur defect	Augmented bone volume and reduced trabecular spacing	[19]
ADSC and PRP	Alginate	Capsules in subcutaneous injection	Greater mineralized tissue volume and mean density of tissue volume	[20]
HDPSC	P_{11}-4	Injected into defect	A lesser extent of osteogenesis and bone remodeling compared to the biomaterial alone	[21]

(continued)

Table 5.1 (continued)

Cell-therapy strategy	Material type	Delivery method	Results and Applications	References
Chondrocytes	RGD-AL/HA	Subcutaneous injection	Stimulated the regeneration of cartilage tissue	[22]
MSC, TGF-β3, and PTHrP	Alginate microcapsules in HA hydrogels	Subcutaneous implants	Neocartilage formation and reduced calcification	[23]
autoC or alloMSC	Alginate	Beads in the knee of each rabbit	Notable cartilage repair	[24]
BMNC	RGDS in PA	Subcutaneous injection	Maintain viability and proliferation of cells	[25]

therapies such as mesenchymal stem cells, induced pluripotent stem cells (iPSCs) and modified cells to secrete angiogenic factors are used to treat post-MI.

Mesenchymal Stem Cells

The mesenchymal stem cell's ability to differentiate into cardiomyocytes was believed to be the primary therapeutic benefit for post-MI regeneration. Research indicates stem cells' release of paracrine factors exerts myocardial protection and repair [31, 32]. An interesting study investigated if the migration of bone marrow-derived mesenchymal stem cells (BMSCs) from the patch into the myocardium or if the paracrine factors released by BMSCs caused the therapeutic effect [16]. After 8 weeks of an MI, rats were administered either human BMSC patch (BMSC-P), BMSCs labeled with iron oxide nanoparticles patch (BMSC*-P), acellular patch (A-P), or were left untreated. When comparing cell tracking T2*-weighted cardiac magnetic resonance measurements of cardiac function post-implantation versus baseline, there was a significant improvement in the two cell-patch treated groups. The BMSC-P group had higher levels of a paracrine factor, fibroblast growth factor-2 (FGF-2), in the infarcted area compared to the control area. Post-infarction LV function was improved, and the paracrine factors of BMSCs were the source of therapy.

MSCs release angiogenic, mitogenic, and anti-inflammatory factors that regulate tissue repair in cardiac diseases [33]. Therefore, clinical trials investigate MSCs to treat myocardial ischemia (NCT01392105, NCT01087996). Many of these clinical trials assessed different delivery methods. For instance, a phase II/III clinical trial found that intracoronary infusion of human BM-derived MSCs had modest improvements in left ventricular ejection fraction (LVEF) [34]. In another phase I/II clinical trial, MSCs were delivered transendocardial, and the patients had improved ventricular remodeling [35]. Unfortunately, in many of these delivery methods, the MSCs had low survival after implantation and thus required new strategies to improve cell survival.

Encapsulating mesenchymal stem cells with biomaterials can help improve cell therapy viability and localization. A triazole-triazole-thiomorpholine dioxide (TMTD) alginate capsules with MSC were implanted in the pericardial sac and found high cell viability after 14 days in vivo [12]. In a post-infarct rat model, at day 28, MSC capsules had more LVEF than MSC injection and blank capsules (Fig. 5.2). MSCs viability can be maintained through biomaterials and sustain the release of paracrine factors to improve ventricular function and remodeling. Interestingly, two delivery methods were used to implant alginate-encapsulated hMSCs with a PEG hydrogel patch to secure the encapsulated hMSCs to the rat-injured myocardium [14]. There was a significant decrease in the scar size after MI with rats treated with encapsulated hMSCs embedded in the gel compared to the other groups. After 28 days, total microvessel density increased in encapsulated hMSCs compared to the other groups. Biomaterials can maintain the MSCs' viability and localize the therapy to maximize the regenerative effect on the site of interest.

Cell engraftment is essential in tissue regeneration. An epicardial placement of MSC dressing was created to retain cell suspension on a coated fibrinogen and thrombin surface, and the alternative side was composed of collagen sheets. [13] The MSC fibrinogen and thrombin-coated side with the MSCs would adhere to the heart surface while the collagen sheets protect the MSC-fibrin complex. After 4 weeks of transplantation of MSCs with the dressing technique or intramyocardial (IM) injection, reduced infarct size was observed in the MSC-dressing therapy and IM injection compared to the sham treatment (Fig. 5.3). MSC dressing had increased neo-vascular formation compared to IM injection.

The biomaterial and delivery method must be compatible with the growth and success of cell-based therapy. An array of biomaterials were compared to see if hMSCs retention would be improved [15]. Five groups were evaluated, saline injection, two injectable hydrogels (alginate and chitosan/B-GP), and two epicardial patches (alginate and collagen). Compared to hearts injected with DiD-GFP hMSCs in saline, alginate and chitosan/B-GP gels showed an eightfold and 14-fold mean increase in fluorescent signal, respectively. An increase in fluorescence was also seen in collagen and alginate patches, which were 47-fold and 59-fold more significant than the saline control. The cells were protected using different biomaterials encapsulation methods, increased viability in hypoxic and ischemic conditions, and retained more cells in the myocardium after 24 hours compared to saline-injected hMSCs.

Induced Pluripotent Stem Cells

Alternative cell sources can be used to reprogram cells with properties similar to embryonic stem cells, such as self-renewal and pluripotency. IPSCs can be a source of therapy without running into ethical issues. They can differentiate into disease-relevant cell types, such as cardiomyocytes, endothelial cells (EC), and smooth muscle cells (SMC). Cardiomyocytes are cells responsible for generating the contraction in the heart. Endothelial cells release substances that control vascular relaxation, contraction, and blood clotting. Smooth muscle cells control blood pressure, distribution and maintains vascular structural

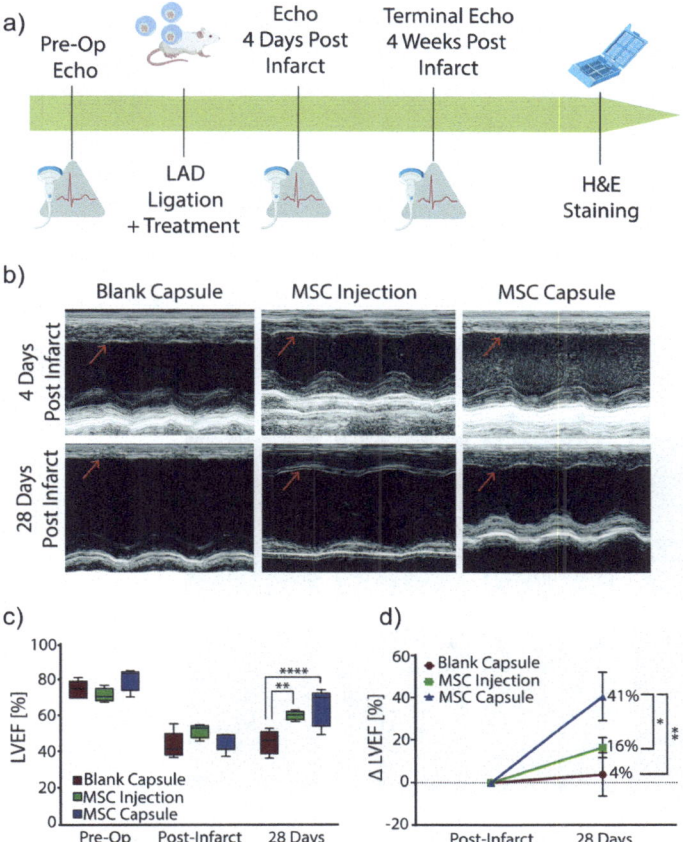

Fig. 5.2 **a** Schematic of the study timeline and endpoint. **b** Representative M-mode echocardiograph images of the papillary muscle 4 days post infarct and 28 days post infarct (n = 4–5). Red arrows identify the left ventricular wall. **c** Left ventricular ejection fraction (LVEF) measurements 1 day prior to infarct, 4 days after, and 28 days (terminal) after acute myocardial infarction (n = 4–5). **d** Delta LVEF plotted to show the improvement in ejection fraction from 4 days post MI to 28 days post MI (terminal) for each group (n = 4–5). % Change was calculated using the formula [(LVEF 28 day (terminal) − LVEF 4-day post-MI)/LVEF 4-day post-MI] × 100. All data are presented as mean ± SEM. *$P < 0.05$, **$P < 0.01$, ****$P < 0.0001$. The figure and caption were reproduced from Biomaterials Science, 2020. [12]

integrity. During an MI, the low supply of blood and oxygen can result in apoptosis and necrosis in the ischemic zone from cardiomyocytes, smooth muscle cells, and endothelial cells. Therefore, CMs have been applied to rodent and non-human primate MI models to replenish the lost cells and found improved cardiac function [36, 37]. A major concern

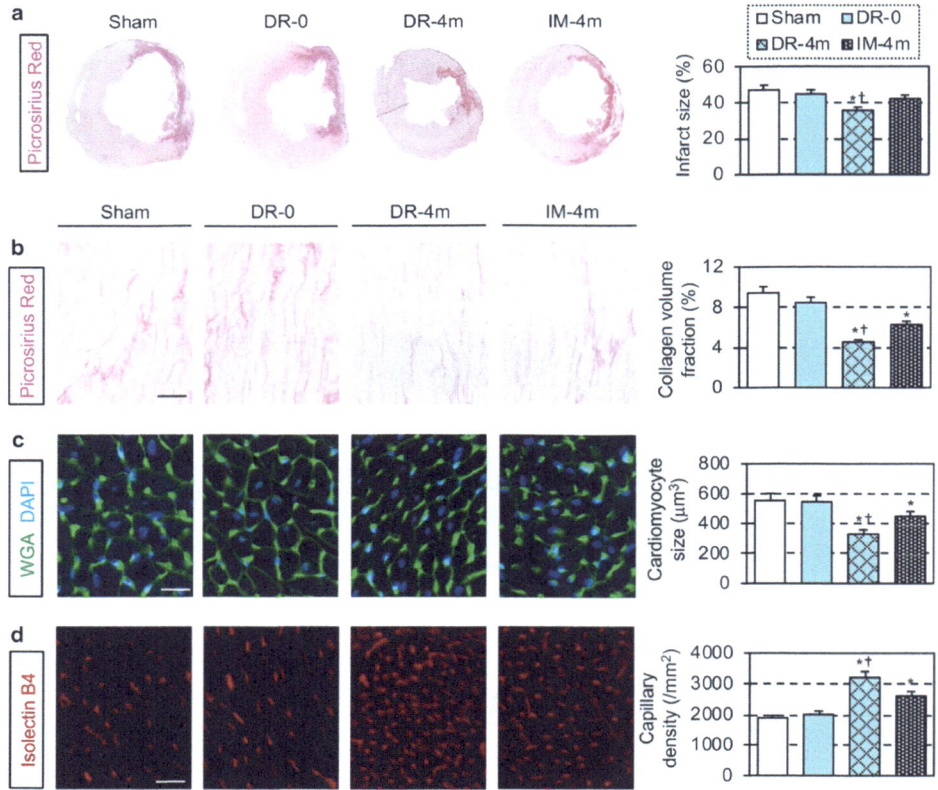

Fig. 5.3 Enhanced repair of the damaged myocardium by MSC-dressing therapy. Heart samples at 4 weeks after transplantation of 4×10^6 rat amnion-derived MSCs (either by MSC-dressing technique or IM injection; DR-4 m and IM-4 m groups, respectively) in a rat ischemic heart failure model were collected and analyzed by histological assessments to elucidate myocardial repair post MSC-based therapy. The DR-0 group received epicardial transplantation of fibrin sealant film only, while the Sham group received no treatment. **a** Representative images of picrosirius red staining of the heart. **b–d** Collagen volume fraction **b**, cardiomyocyte hypertrophy (**c**) and capillary density **d** in the peri-infarct viable myocardium measured using heart samples stained with/for picrosirius red, wheat germ agglutinin and isolectin B4, respectively. n = 5 in each group, *$P < 0.05$ vs. Sham and DR-0 groups, †$P < 0.05$ vs. IM-4 m group. One-way ANOVA. Scale bars = 100 μm (**b, d**) and 25 μm (**c**). (For interpretation of the references to color in this figure legend, the reader is referred to the Web version of this article.) The figure and caption were reproduced from Biomaterials, 2019 [13]

with the delivery of CMs is that in non-human primate models of MI, experienced ventricular arrhythmias must be addressed before widely applying it to the clinic [38]. Like many delivered cells, cardiomyocytes must be locally retained for maximum therapeutic benefit.

Encapsulating hiPSCs-derived cell types with biomaterials can help improve regeneration after an MI. A fibrin scaffold loaded with hiPSCs, deriving CMs, endothelial cells, and smooth muscle cells, with loaded thrombin to form a human cardiac muscle patch (hCMP) [17]. A porcine model treated with either hCMPs upon MI, cell-free open fibrin patches upon MI, neither experiment patch upon MI, or sham surgery. hCMP significantly improved LVF, infarct size, and myocardial wall stress (Fig. 5.4).

Modified Cells
Modified cells can be used to secrete the therapeutic factor and treat MI. Chinese hamster ovary (CHO) cells were genetically modified to secrete VEGF in alginate-poly-L-lysine-alginate (APA) microcapsules [18]. Post-MI, surviving rats were administered microcapsule-CHO (MC-CHO), CHO, blank microcapsule, and culture medium without serum. After 3 weeks of transplantation, there was a decline in fractional shortening and LV enlargement in the MC-CHO group, which was notably lower compared to the other groups. Additionally, the MC-CHO group's therapeutic angiogenic effect significantly increased compared to all three groups. The microencapsulated cells' survival after implantation was maintained, protected xenogeneic cells from immune rejection, and recovered heart function. Using biomaterials as a delivery vehicle for cell-based therapies is beneficial and has inexhaustible treatment applications.

5.3 Tissue Regeneration

Tissue regeneration is the restoration of damaged tissues, organs, and body parts to regain function. Cell therapy has served as a basis for tissue engineering and regeneration. For instance, the FDA has approved using Carticel, autologous chondrocytes, to treat focal articular cartilage defects. These autologous chondrocytes, like many autologous cells, need to be harvested from the patient, expanded ex vivo, and implanted at the injury site. This delays treatment compared to allogeneic cell sources with low antigenicity and can be mass-produced with minimal risk of an adverse event. In many cases, the cells require support structures that can be achieved with biomaterials and can be loaded with growth factors to promote regeneration. Biomaterial-based cell therapies have used human bone marrow stromal cells (HBMSC), human dental pulp stromal cells (HDP-SCs), adipose-derived stem cells (ADSC), and platelet-rich plasma (PRP), bone marrow mononuclear cells (BMNC), chondrocytes, and MSCs in tissue regeneration applications. There are several avenues tissue regeneration is applied, such as bone regeneration, cartilage regeneration, and ischemic tissue disease.

Bone Regeneration
Bone regeneration is the physiological process of forming bone during healing and remodeling throughout life. Bone health can be affected by osteoporosis, the development of

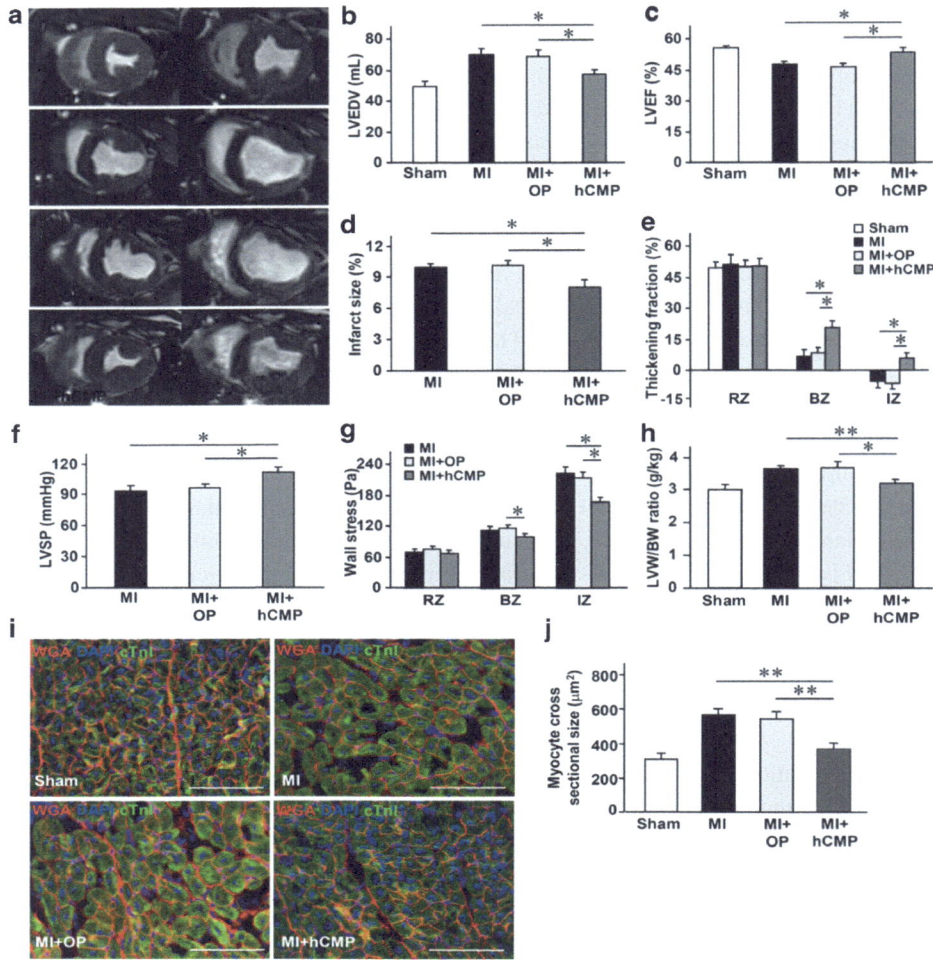

◀**Fig. 5.4** hCMP transplantation improves the recovery of cardiac function and limits adverse remodeling in infarcted pig hearts. MI was surgically induced in swine hearts by occluding the coronary artery for 60 min; then, 2 hCMPs were sutured over the site of infarction in animals from the MI + hCMP group, 2 large fibrin patches lacking the hiPSC-derived cardiac cells were sutured over the injury site in animals from the MI + OP group, and animals in the MI group recovered without either experimental treatment. Animals in the Sham group underwent all surgical procedures for MI induction, with the exception of the occlusion step. **a** through **e** Four weeks after MI or Sham surgery, magnetic resonance images **a** (Left, end systole; Right, end diastole) were obtained and used to measure left ventricular end-diastolic volumes (LVEDV) **b**, left ventricular ejection fractions (LVEF) **c** infarct sizes **d** and systolic thickening fractions **e** in the infarcted zone (IZ) of the LV wall, in the border zone (BZ) of the infarct, and in a remote (ie, noninfarcted) zone (RZ). n = 8 to 10 per experimental group. **f**, Hemodynamic measurements. **g** End-systolic LV wall stress in the IZ, BZ, and RZ. n = 5 to 7 per experimental group. **h** through **j** Animals were euthanized at week 4; then, the LV weight to body weight (LVW/BW) ratios were determined (n = 8–11 per experimental group) **h**. **i** and **j** Sections from the border zone of the infarct were collected and stained with wheat germ agglutinin (WGA) and cTnI to visualize cardiomyocytes (n = 6–8 per experimental group, scale bar = 100 μm) **i**. Nuclei were counterstained with DAPI, and cardiomyocyte cross-sectional surface areas were measured **j**. *$P < 0.05$. **$P < 0.01$. cTnI indicates cardiac troponin I; DAPI, 4′,6-diamidino-2-phenylindole; hCMP, human cardiac muscle patch; hiPSC, human induced-pluripotent stem cell; LV, left ventricle; MI, myocardial infarction; and OP, open fibrin patches. The figure and caption were reproduced from Circulation, 2017 [17]

cancer, and infections. Traditional medicine utilizes distraction osteogenesis and bone transport, which are technically demanding techniques [39]. Bone grafting is a standard surgical procedure to promote bone regeneration. One of the types of bone grafts applies autologous bone, which combines osteoinduction, osteogenesis, and osteoconduction. Another type of bone graft is allogenic bone, such as demineralized bone matrix, morselized and cancellous chips, and whole-bone segments, which can be employed depending on the patient site requirements. Allogenic bone grafts have reduced bone morphogenetic proteins (BMPs) and other growth factors without cellular components. Therefore, tissue engineering strategies such as scaffolds utilize biomaterials for bone reconstruction as their porosity and mechanical properties can be altered to mimic bone architecture [40]. In addition to biomaterial scaffold ability, cells are loaded for additional healing properties. Some cells loaded in biomaterials used in bone regeneration are HBMSC, HDPSCs, ADSCs, and PRPs.

Encapsulated cell-based therapies offer increased angiogenesis, temporal regulation, and coordination of signal cascades, essential factors that stimulate bone regeneration. A scaffold was constructed to co-deliver BMP-2 in alginate and poly($_{D,L}$-lactic acid) (PLA) to slow the rate of release and VEGF$_{165}$ in alginate fibers to accelerate the rate of release [19]. HBMSCs were transplanted onto the alginate-VEGF$_{155}$/P$_{DL}$LA-BMP-2 scaffolds to investigate bone regeneration capacity. After 28 days of implantation, nude mice with segmental femur defect treated with alginate-VEGF$_{165}$/P$_{DL}$LA-BMP-2 seeded with HBMSCs alginate displayed increased bone volume and reduced trabecular spacing. Histological examination confirmed that extensive collagen matrix deposition was found only in alginate-VEGF$_{165}$/P$_{DL}$LA-BMP-2 seeded with HBMSCs. Osteoid formation within the defect region was found in all the groups, but only alginate-VEGF$_{165}$/P$_{DL}$LA-BMP-2 seeded with HBMSCs had evidence of mineralized collagen. Extensive bone remodeling was seen through increased tartrate-resistant acid phosphatase in alginate-VEGF$_{165}$/P$_{DL}$LA-BMP-2 seeded with HBMSCs. Using biomaterial scaffolds with cell therapy and combining them with angiogenic and osteogenic factors stimulates bone regeneration.

Combining different cell-based therapies can offer osteogenic and angiogenic potential for bone regeneration. ADSC and PRP from rabbits were encapsulated in alginate and found to enhance vascularization and mineralization in vivo [20]. ADSCs have comparable multilineage capacity to BMSCs but can be harvested at high yield and have less invasive procedures. Additionally, activated PRPs can secrete various growth factors such as VEGF, angiopoietin, and platelet-derived growth factors, ultimately having a continuous supply of growth factors for bone regeneration [41]. After the 1-month and 3-month time points, nude mice treated with either 10% PRP-ADSC-laden or 15% PRP-ADSC-laden microcapsules presented a white calcified matrix compared to the other three groups. Micro-CT analysis of the heterotopic bone formation at 3 months showed that the percentage of mineralized tissue volume was significantly greater in 15% PRP-ADSC-laden microcapsules (Fig. 5.5). Histology quantitative analysis demonstrated that 10% PRP-ADSC-laden and 15% PRP-ADSC-laden microcapsules microvascular densities were considerably higher than the other groups. Both microcapsule groups enhanced vascularization and mineralization to incite bone regeneration.

Including cell-based therapies in biomaterials can alter the porosity and mechanical structure of the biomaterial as a scaffold. HDPSCs can be accessed by harvesting the pulp from the teeth [42–44]. HDPSCs have shown proliferative and multilineage differentiation potential [43]. Therefore, HDPSCs' qualities can be a source of bone regeneration. HDPSCs were sequestered using clinically available self-assembling peptide, P$_{11}$-4 (P$_{11}$-4 + HDPSCs) [21]. Interestingly, P$_{11}$-4 + HDPSCs did not accelerate bone repair compared to P$_{11}$-4 alone. P$_{11}$-4 alone degraded slower and was, therefore, suitable to support osteogenesis and bone remodeling compared to P$_{11}$-4 + HDPSCs. Thus, it is crucial to consider the biologics incorporated into biomaterials can ultimately affect the degradation rate. Cell-based therapies in biomaterials can serve valuable in bone regeneration as long as the scaffold structure remains intact and supports the site-directed delivery of therapeutic factors.

Cartilage Regeneration
Cartilage regeneration aims to restore the flexible connective tissue between joints and bones for smooth motion. Cartilage can be damaged in various ways, such as osteoarthritis, trauma, or osteonecrosis. The current surgical options for partial cartilage lesions are microfracture and autologous chondrocyte implantation. For complete cartilage degeneration, total joint replacement is needed. Therefore, cartilage tissue engineering strategies are required to provide the appropriate environment for cell growth and chondrogenic

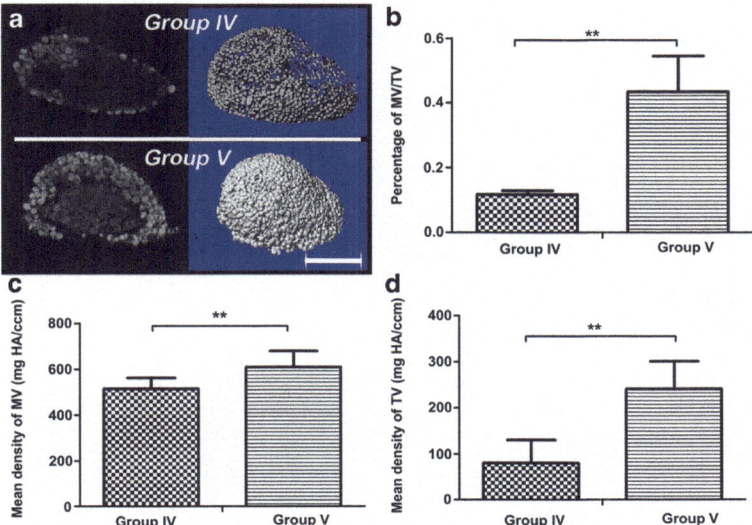

Fig. 5.5 Micro-CT analysis of the heterotopic bone formation of 10% PRP-ADSC-laden (group IV) and 15% PRP-ADSC-laden microspheres (group V) at 3 months. **a** three-dimensional and cross-sectional images of the implants, scale bar is 2 mm **b** percentage of mineralized tissue volume, **c** mean density of mineralized volume, and **d** mean density of tissue volume (*$P < 0.05$, **$P < 0.01$, ***$P < 0.001$). The figure and caption were reprinted after permission from Biomaterials, 2012 [20]

differentiation. Cell therapies such as chondrocytes and MSCs are being used to regenerate cartilage. An essential function of chondrocytes is the production of extracellular matrix (ECM) proteins which lubricate the surface of joints and bones [45–47]. MSCs can differentiate into fibroblasts and chondrocytes in cartilage, ultimately aiding in the increased accumulation of proteoglycans. In conjunction, biomaterials and cells can mimic the cartilage ECM needed for regeneration.

Biomaterials can incorporate peptides to promote interactions with chondrocytes and have cartilage regeneration. An alginate formulation with RGD, a cell adhesion-promoting bioactive amino acid sequence, and hyaluronate hydrogels (RGD-AL/HA) stimulated the regeneration of cartilage tissue when treated with primary chondrocytes [22]. Quantitative analysis of collagen type II expression in tissues was significantly higher in nude mice treated with primary chondrocytes with RGD-AL/HA compared to the other three groups. Histological analysis showed that the RGD-AL/HA gels effectively formed ECM, demonstrated by the large number of sulfated glycosaminoglycans (GAGs) in newly formed tissues (Fig. 5.6). Chondrogenic gene expression showed that RGD-AL/HA had the highest levels of aggrecan, collagen type II, and SOX-9 gene expression compared to the other

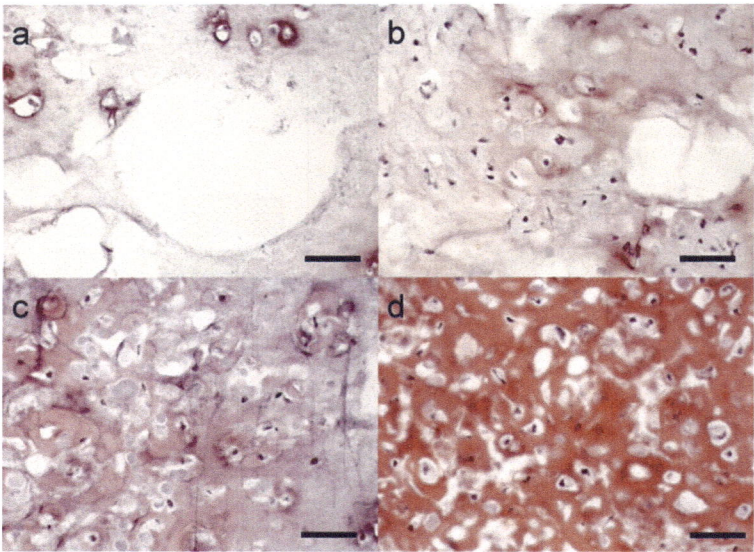

Fig. 5.6 Images of Safranin-O-stained tissue sections retrieved from mice (scale bar, 50 μm). Cells were transplanted with **a** media only, **b** non-modified alginate, **c** RGD-modified alginate, and **d** RGD-modified alginate/hyaluronate. The figure and caption were reprinted after permission from Carbohydrate Polymers, 2011. [22]

groups. The expression of these characteristics are important factors that contribute to cartilage regeneration since they are either structural components expressed in all cartilage tissue or directly influence the collagen type II gene.

Co-delivery of cells and growth factors in biomaterials can aid in cartilage regeneration. Parathyroid hormone-related protein (PTHrP) was co-delivered to reduce calcification in MSC-laden nanofilm-coated HA hydrogels and determined if transforming growth factor-β3 (TGF-β3) loaded microcapsules improved cartilage regeneration [23]. From the 4-week and the 8-week time point, there was an increase in mechanical stiffness in nude mice treated with TGF-β3 microcapsules and microcapsules with both TGF-β3 and PTHrP. Microcapsules with TGF-β3 and PTHrP showed higher GAG content than the other two groups. Calcium content in microcapsules with TGF-β3 and PTHrP decreased compared to microcapsules with only TGF-β3. A single dose of TGF-β3 in nanofilm-coated alginate microcapsules encapsulated in HA hydrogels stimulating chondrogenesis of encapsulated MSCs, resulted in the neocartilage formation and reduction of calcification by co-delivering PTHrP.

Cells have unique functions which may impact cartilage regeneration differently. Autologous chondrocytes (autoC) or allogeneic undifferentiated MSC (alloMSC) were compared in alginate beads to determine which cell type had greater cartilage regeneration in rats [24]. After 6 months, quantitative morphological observations showed that alloMSCs and autoC had more cartilage tissue regeneration than the untreated group. Quantitative histology of regenerated cartilage tissue and GAG concentrations are significantly higher in treated groups than in controls. There was not a significant difference between the alloMSC and autoC groups. Both alloMSCs and autoC had notable cartilage repair.

Ischemic Tissue Disease

Ischemic tissue disease occurs when the supply does not match the tissue demand for oxygen. The reduced blood flow can cause tissue damage and can be irreversible if the blood flow is not restored. Once the blood flow is reestablished, it can recover cells and, paradoxically, in ischemic tissue, can have reperfusion injury. Several organs, like the brain, heart, kidney, and liver, are susceptible to ischemia. Therefore, it is crucial to address the regeneration of ischemic tissue. Biomaterials can locally retain and maintain transplanted cells' viability within ischemic tissue, which is necessary to improve the efficacy of cell-based therapies.

The regenerative potential of cell-based therapies has been applied in ischemic tissue disease. Endothelial progenitor cells, precursors of mature endothelial cells, mobilize from the bone marrow and home to the ischemic zone, where they repair ischemic tissue [48]. BMNCs induce this regeneration but require local retention and high viability for maximal regenerative effect [49]. Therefore, RGDS was incorporated into PA as a delivery vehicle for BMNC [25]. In vivo bioluminescent imaging showed transplanted luciferase-expressing BMNCs in RGDS PA maintained the highest bioluminescent signal compared to all other groups (Fig. 5.7). Using biomaterials as a delivery vehicle can maintain viability and promote the proliferation of cells.

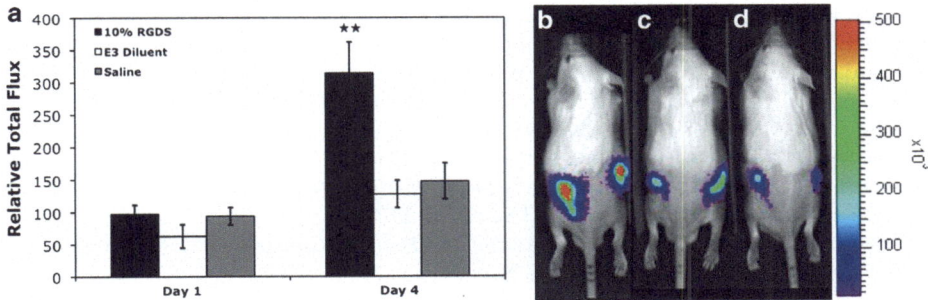

Fig. 5.7 Quantification from in vivo bioluminescent imaging of transplanted luciferase-expressing BMNCs **a** injected subcutaneously, encapsulated within the binary RGDS system (**b**, $n = 15$) and E3 diluent PA (**c**, $n = 11$), along with a saline control (**d**, $n = 13$). ** $P < 0.01$. The figure and caption were reprinted after permission from Acta Biomaterialia, 2010 [25]

5.4 Conclusions

Cell-based therapies are versatile living drugs that can be tailored to therapeutic applications. Cells can be used inherently or modified to secrete therapeutic factors in myocardial infarction and tissue regenerative strategies. Clinically, cellular therapeutics have failed due to complications in retaining and maintaining cell viability at the site of interest. Biomaterials can overcome these barriers as they can locally control the release of the cellular therapeutic. A consideration of cell-based therapies is the biomaterial's rapid degradation, which can expose the cells to the external environment, resulting in an immune response towards the therapeutic and unwanted side effects [7, 50]. It is imperative to find the optimal time point in ensuring the dosage of the cell therapeutic is delivered and remains local to the delivery site. Aside from myocardial infarction and tissue regeneration, these cell-based therapies in biomaterials hold promise in various other applications.

References

1. Heathman, T.R., et al., *The translation of cell-based therapies: clinical landscape and manufacturing challenges.* Regen Med, 2015. **10**(1): p. 49-64.
2. El-Kadiry, A.E., M. Rafei, and R. Shammaa, *Cell Therapy: Types, Regulation, and Clinical Benefits.* Front Med (Lausanne), 2021. **8**: p. 756029.
3. Basile, G., et al., *Emerging diabetes therapies: Bringing back the beta-cells.* Mol Metab, 2022. **60**: p. 101477.
4. Wang, Q., et al., *The Effect of Schwann Cells/Schwann Cell-Like Cells on Cell Therapy for Peripheral Neuropathy.* Front Cell Neurosci, 2022. **16**: p. 836931.
5. Mu, L., R. Dong, and B. Guo, *Biomaterials-Based Cell Therapy for Myocardial Tissue Regeneration.* Adv Healthc Mater, 2023. **12**(10): p. e2202699.
6. Solazzo, M., et al., *The rationale and emergence of electroconductive biomaterial scaffolds in cardiac tissue engineering.* APL Bioeng, 2019. **3**(4): p. 041501.
7. Sedighi, M., et al., *Therapeutic bacteria to combat cancer; current advances, challenges, and opportunities.* Cancer Med, 2019. **8**(6): p. 3167-3181.
8. Ikada, Y., *Challenges in tissue engineering.* J R Soc Interface, 2006. **3**(10): p. 589-601.
9. Yang, F., et al., *Injectable and redox-responsive hydrogel with adaptive degradation rate for bone regeneration.* J Mater Chem B, 2014. **2**(3): p. 295-304.
10. Chaudhari, A.A., et al., *Future Prospects for Scaffolding Methods and Biomaterials in Skin Tissue Engineering: A Review.* Int J Mol Sci, 2016. **17**(12).
11. Hitscherich, P., et al., *Injectable Self-Assembling Peptide Hydrogels for Tissue Writing and Embryonic Stem Cell Culture.* J Biomed Nanotechnol, 2018. **14**(4): p. 802-807.
12. Ghanta, R.K., et al., *Immune-modulatory alginate protects mesenchymal stem cells for sustained delivery of reparative factors to ischemic myocardium.* Biomater Sci, 2020. **8**(18): p. 5061-5070.
13. Kobayashi, K., et al., *On-site fabrication of Bi-layered adhesive mesenchymal stromal cell-dressings for the treatment of heart failure.* Biomaterials, 2019. **209**: p. 41-53.
14. Levit, R.D., et al., *Cellular encapsulation enhances cardiac repair.* J Am Heart Assoc, 2013. **2**(5): p. e000367.

15. Roche, E.T., et al., *Comparison of biomaterial delivery vehicles for improving acute retention of stem cells in the infarcted heart.* Biomaterials, 2014. **35**(25): p. 6850-6858.
16. Blondiaux, E., et al., *Bone marrow-derived mesenchymal stem cell-loaded fibrin patches act as a reservoir of paracrine factors in chronic myocardial infarction.* J Tissue Eng Regen Med, 2017. **11**(12): p. 3417-3427.
17. Gao, L., et al., *Large Cardiac Muscle Patches Engineered From Human Induced-Pluripotent Stem Cell-Derived Cardiac Cells Improve Recovery From Myocardial Infarction in Swine.* Circulation, 2018. **137**(16): p. 1712-1730.
18. Zhang, H., et al., *Transplantation of microencapsulated genetically modified xenogeneic cells augments angiogenesis and improves heart function.* Gene Ther, 2008. **15**(1): p. 40-8.
19. Kanczler, J.M., et al., *The effect of the delivery of vascular endothelial growth factor and bone morphogenic protein-2 to osteoprogenitor cell populations on bone formation.* Biomaterials, 2010. **31**(6): p. 1242-50.
20. Man, Y., et al., *Angiogenic and osteogenic potential of platelet-rich plasma and adipose-derived stem cell laden alginate microspheres.* Biomaterials, 2012. **33**(34): p. 8802-11.
21. Saha, S., et al., *A biomimetic self-assembling peptide promotes bone regeneration in vivo: A rat cranial defect study.* Bone, 2019. **127**: p. 602-611.
22. Honghyun Park, K.Y.L., *Facile control of RGD-alginate/hyaluronate hydrogel formation for cartilage regeneration.* Carbohydrate Polymers, 2011. **86**(3): p. 1107–1112.
23. Bian, L., et al., *Enhanced MSC chondrogenesis following delivery of TGF-beta3 from alginate microspheres within hyaluronic acid hydrogels in vitro and in vivo.* Biomaterials, 2011. **32**(27): p. 6425-34.
24. Tay, L.X., et al., *Treatment outcomes of alginate-embedded allogenic mesenchymal stem cells versus autologous chondrocytes for the repair of focal articular cartilage defects in a rabbit model.* Am J Sports Med, 2012. **40**(1): p. 83-90.
25. Webber, M.J., et al., *Development of bioactive peptide amphiphiles for therapeutic cell delivery.* Acta Biomater, 2010. **6**(1): p. 3-11.
26. Ibanez, B., et al., *2017 ESC Guidelines for the management of acute myocardial infarction in patients presenting with ST-segment elevation: The Task Force for the management of acute myocardial infarction in patients presenting with ST-segment elevation of the European Society of Cardiology (ESC).* Eur Heart J, 2018. **39**(2): p. 119-177.
27. Lu, L., et al., *Myocardial Infarction: Symptoms and Treatments.* Cell Biochem Biophys, 2015. **72**(3): p. 865-7.
28. Roffi, M., et al., *2015 ESC Guidelines for the management of acute coronary syndromes in patients presenting without persistent ST-segment elevation: Task Force for the Management of Acute Coronary Syndromes in Patients Presenting without Persistent ST-Segment Elevation of the European Society of Cardiology (ESC).* Eur Heart J, 2016. **37**(3): p. 267-315.
29. Heusch, G., et al., *Cardiovascular remodelling in coronary artery disease and heart failure.* Lancet, 2014. **383**(9932): p. 1933-43.
30. Zornoff, L.A., et al., *Ventricular remodeling after myocardial infarction: concepts and clinical implications.* Arq Bras Cardiol, 2009. **92**(2): p. 150-64.
31. Gnecchi, M., et al., *Paracrine action accounts for marked protection of ischemic heart by Akt-modified mesenchymal stem cells.* Nat Med, 2005. **11**(4): p. 367-8.
32. Yoshioka, T., et al., *Repair of infarcted myocardium mediated by transplanted bone marrow-derived CD34+ stem cells in a nonhuman primate model.* Stem Cells, 2005. **23**(3): p. 355-64.
33. Pankajakshan, D. and D.K. Agrawal, *Mesenchymal Stem Cell Paracrine Factors in Vascular Repair and Regeneration.* J Biomed Technol Res, 2014. **1**(1).

34. Lee, J.W., et al., *A randomized, open-label, multicenter trial for the safety and efficacy of adult mesenchymal stem cells after acute myocardial infarction.* J Korean Med Sci, 2014. **29**(1): p. 23-31.
35. Hare, J.M., et al., *Comparison of allogeneic vs autologous bone marrow-derived mesenchymal stem cells delivered by transendocardial injection in patients with ischemic cardiomyopathy: the POSEIDON randomized trial.* JAMA, 2012. **308**(22): p. 2369-79.
36. Riegler, J., et al., *Human Engineered Heart Muscles Engraft and Survive Long Term in a Rodent Myocardial Infarction Model.* Circ Res, 2015. **117**(8): p. 720-30.
37. Shiba, Y., et al., *Allogeneic transplantation of iPS cell-derived cardiomyocytes regenerates primate hearts.* Nature, 2016. **538**(7625): p. 388-391.
38. Chong, J.J., et al., *Human embryonic-stem-cell-derived cardiomyocytes regenerate non-human primate hearts.* Nature, 2014. **510**(7504): p. 273-7.
39. Dimitriou, R., et al., *Bone regeneration: current concepts and future directions.* BMC Med, 2011. **9**: p. 66.
40. Gong, T., et al., *Nanomaterials and bone regeneration.* Bone Res, 2015. **3**: p. 15029.
41. Intini, G., *The use of platelet-rich plasma in bone reconstruction therapy.* Biomaterials, 2009. **30**(28): p. 4956-66.
42. Gronthos, S., et al., *Postnatal human dental pulp stem cells (DPSCs) <i>in vitro</i> and <i>in</i> <i>vivo</i>.* Proceedings of the National Academy of Sciences, 2000. **97**(25): p. 13625-13630.
43. Leyendecker Junior, A., et al., *The use of human dental pulp stem cells for in vivo bone tissue engineering: A systematic review.* J Tissue Eng, 2018. **9**: p. 2041731417752766.
44. Yamada, Y., et al., *A feasibility of useful cell-based therapy by bone regeneration with deciduous tooth stem cells, dental pulp stem cells, or bone-marrow-derived mesenchymal stem cells for clinical study using tissue engineering technology.* Tissue Eng Part A, 2010. **16**(6): p. 1891-900.
45. Greene, G.W., et al., *Adaptive mechanically controlled lubrication mechanism found in articular joints.* Proc Natl Acad Sci U S A, 2011. **108**(13): p. 5255-9.
46. Nam, Y., et al., *Current Therapeutic Strategies for Stem Cell-Based Cartilage Regeneration.* Stem Cells Int, 2018. **2018**: p. 8490489.
47. Sophia Fox, A.J., A. Bedi, and S.A. Rodeo, *The basic science of articular cartilage: structure, composition, and function.* Sports Health, 2009. **1**(6): p. 461-8.
48. Asahara, T., et al., *Bone marrow origin of endothelial progenitor cells responsible for postnatal vasculogenesis in physiological and pathological neovascularization.* Circ Res, 1999. **85**(3): p. 221-8.
49. Balsam, L.B., et al., *Haematopoietic stem cells adopt mature haematopoietic fates in ischaemic myocardium.* Nature, 2004. **428**(6983): p. 668-73.
50. Fischbach, M.A., J.A. Bluestone, and W.A. Lim, *Cell-based therapeutics: the next pillar of medicine.* Sci Transl Med, 2013. **5**(179): p. 179ps7.

Recent Clinical Trials on Immunomodulatory Biomaterials Applications

Sudip Mukherjee

6.1 Clinical Trials

Various technologies related to immunomodulatory biomaterials were under clinical trials recently and are being explored to transition them from laboratory to bench-side. Some of these trials have demonstrated huge potential in cell-based therapy, drug delivery and other biomedical implants for the treatment of cancer, diabetes, tissue regeneration etc. (Table 6.1). Use of these innovative biomaterials for delivery of cells, drugs or material itself has changed the dynamics of modern therapy observed by the significant changes in the recent clinical trials. In this section we will briefly discuss the different clinical trials and their current status.

The most significant development in the field of cell therapy happened with the recent FDA approval of Lantidra, which is infusion of allogenic pancreatic beta islets to the portal vein of human liver affected with type 1 diabetes (T1D). The technology developed by CellTrans is innovative and transformative [2]. In another similar strategy by Vertex for their VX-880, an infused allogeneic stem cell-derived insulin-producing islet cells. Even though both technologies are remarkable in developing solutions for treating many T1D affected patients, they are not long-term as the majority of the patients require doses of insulin within 12–60 months following first doses. Apart from that they may also require chronic immunosuppressive therapy making the patients vulnerable to potential side-effects and development of auto immunity. Hence, technologies that can utilize immune protection are the solution to prevent cell graft loss and long-term therapy.

S. Mukherjee (✉)
School of Biomedical Engineering, Indian Institute of Technology (BHU), Varanasi 221005, UP, India
e-mail: sudip.bme@iitbhu.ac.in

Table 6.1 Current examples of clinical trials of different immunomodulatory biomaterials. The table is reproduced and modified following permissions from Wiley [1]

Company/Institution	Cell type	Material	Treatment	Phase	National Clinical Trial number (NCT)
Diatranz Otsuka Limited	Neonatal Porcine Islets encapsulated in alginate	Alginate capsules	T1D	I/II, I/II, II	NCT00940173, NCT01739829, NCT01736228
Sigilon Therapeutics, Eli Lilly	iPSC-derived islet cell therapy encapsuled in immunoprotected alginate microcapsules	Small molecule modified alginate microcapsules.SIG-002	T1D	Preclinical	–
Uppsala University Hospital	Islets encapsulated to alginate hydrogel in combination with a Gas Chamber	Alginate-based Hydrogel	T1D	I/II	NCT02064309
Via Cyte	Pancreatic Progenitor cells in an implantable device/or without device	PEC-Encap™ (VC-01™)/ PEC-Direct™ (VC-02™)	T1D	I/II, I	NCT02239354, NCT02939118, NCT03162926
Vertex	Stem cell derived differentiated pancreatic beta cells		T1D		–
Avenge Bio and Rice University	Polymeric microcapsules containing therapeutic cells using LOCOcyte™	AVB-001	Metastatic peritoneal cancer		NCT05538624
Maxivax SA	MVX-1	MVX-ONCO-1	Cancer	I	NCT02193503
Assistance Publique—Hôpitaux de Paris	Human Embryonic Stem Cells-derived CD15 + Isl-1 + progenitors	Fibrin Patch	Ischemic Heart Disease	I	NCT02057900

(continued)

Table 6.1 (continued)

Company/Institution	Cell type	Material	Treatment	Phase	National Clinical Trial number (NCT)
Bellerophon (Bellerophon BCM LLC)	–	IK-5001	MI	I/II	NCT00557531, NCT01226563
Lone Star Heart, Inc	–	Calcium-Alginate Hydrogel	Dilated Cardiomyopathy, HF	II, II/III	NCT00847964, NCT01311791, NCT03082508
University Medical Center Utrecht	Allogeneic Mesenchymal Stem Cells and Autologous Chondrons	Fibrin Glue	Cartilage Damage	I/II, III	NCT02037204, NCT04236739
Biosolution Co., Ltd	Autologous Chondrocytes	Cartilife®	Articular Cartilage Lesion of Knee	I, II	NCT03517046, NCT03545269

ViaCyte in collaboration with Diatranz Otsuka Limited and Uppsala University Hospital developed DIABECELL®, a transplantable cell therapy-based technology utilizing immunoprotective alginate microcapsules containing xenogeneic porcine islets for the cure of T1D. Even with xenogeneic cells it the therapy showed remarkable success in reducing hyperglycemia, HbA1C levels and abnormal hypoglycemia in the nighttime when tested in the Phase I/II clinical studies (NCT00940173). Intraperitoneal (IP) doses of 5,000 IEQ/kg to 20,000 IEQ/kg islets were utilized for the treatment of human patients. In recent developments Eli Lilly has acquired a Boston based company named Sigilon Therapeutics for iPSC-derived islet cell therapy encapsulated in immunoprotected alginate microcapsules 'SIG-002' [2]. The immunoprotected hydrogels are developed using the technology of Vegas and Veiseh published in Nature Biotechnology [3]. This brings a giant player like Eli Lilly to this exciting space of research.

In another clinical trial (NCT02064309), Beta-O_2 Technologies Ltd. in collaboration with Uppsala University Hospital developed a microdevice containing human beta islets and are currently undergoing phase I/II studies. The transplantable device containing human islets were instrumental to reduce hyperglycemia when tested in four different patients. Moreover, the therapy was able to reduce the occurrence of abnormal hypoglycemia, infection, fibrosis and local inflammation around the device even after 3 months. The technology works to oxygenate the cells to keep them alive for long-term therapy. One out of four patients had a detectable level of C-peptide even after 3 months of implantation of the therapeutic device [4]. Three patients had a corrected level of HbA1c, but were statistically insignificant.

ViaCyte has developed another few remarkable technologies PEC-Direct™ (VC-02™) and PEC-Encap™ (VC-01™) that used stem cell-derived pancreatic progenitor cells in immunoprotective implantable devices. VC-01™ are protected by an immunomodulatory layer to protect the inner cells against invading immune cell attack, but granting the access of nutrients and oxygens that are needed for the prolonged cell survival. Currently several phase I/II clinical trials are undergoing using these technologies for testing the efficacy of the transplantation and having a long-term glycemic control for the treatment of T1D (NCT02239354; NCT02939118). VC-02™ contains a layer of polymer coating around the cells enabling rapid vascularization of transplanted cells. Moreover, this treatment is implanted under the skin. Rapid vascularization allows the cells to get access to sufficient oxygen and nutrients, important for long-term cell survival and successful therapy. Phase I clinical trials are currently undergoing to test the safety of these devices for four months in patients having T1D where they will get transplantation of up to six devices of PEC-01 (NCT03162926).

Various recent research is ongoing to develop cell-based therapies using immunoprotective biomaterials for cancers. In an exciting new development Avenge Bio and Rice University is currently performing Phase I/II clinical trial using their immunotherapy platform (AVB-001). AVB-001 contains genetically engineered cells secreting interleukin-2 cytokine encapsulated in immunoprotective polymers. Currently clinical trials are undergoing for the treatment of refractory ovarian cancer and evaluating the toxicity profiles (NCT05538624). Moreover, Avenge Bio recently obtained orphan drug status for AVB-001 from FDA on its advance strategies for pleural malignant mesothelioma. In another recent development, Maxivax SA designed and made MVX-ONCO that is used to subcutaneously deliver microcapsules containing genetically engineered allogeneic cells secreting huGM-CSF. Safety evaluation was performed in Phase-I clinical studies using six doses of MVX-ONCO-1 that was implanted subcutaneously to patients suffering from late staged metastatic solid tumor (NCT02193503). Four patients out of six demonstrated positive outcome of the therapy with lesser tumor burden, and better survival. The capsules were retrieved following seven days to confirm the steady production of huGM-CSF [5].

Cardiovascular disease prognosis has seen remarkable discoveries and interventions utilizing immunomodulatory biomaterials in recent years. Assistance Publique—Hôpitaux de Paris developed a therapeutic fibrin-based patch containing human embryonic stem cells for treating diseases related to ischemic heart. Phase-I study results demonstrated six out of six participants has an improved wall motion of the heart when treated with therapeutic fibrin patch loaded with human stem cells in a timely manner (NCT02057900). Following one year of the therapeutic implants, participants had an elevation in LV ejection fraction (LVEF) and minor reduction in LV volumes, with no time dependent significance [6].

Bellerophon therapeutics created a bioabsorbable scaffold (IK-5001), an intracoronary injection of a mixture of 0.3% calcium gluconate and 1% sodium alginate (IK-5001) for the treatment of left ventricular (LV) restoration following myocardial infarction (MI) [7]. IK-5001 therapy following 7 days of MI has restored various notable clinical parameters including LVEF, LV end-systolic and end-diastolic volume indexes after six months in their Phase-I clinical trial conducted in 27 participants (NCT00557531). NT-proBNP, a cardiovascular biomarker was related to heart failure was reduced confirming the utility of the biomaterials therapy. In another of their clinical trial patients were injected a varying volume of treatments (±4 mL) showing better performance in the 6-min walk test (6MWT) without a statistical significance (NCT01226563) [8]. Compared to the sham saline group, biomaterials scaffold treatment (IK-5001) has helped in the improvement of LV end-diastolic volume indexes (LVEDVI) from baseline following six months of the therapy with reduced deaths.

LoneStar Heart, Inc. developed Algisyl-LVR a calcium-alginate crosslinked hydrogel, for the treatment of dilated cardiomyopathy [9]. Improved LV wall thickness was observed in three participants, following the implantation of Algisyl-LVR in a Phase II clinical trial confirmed using a coronary artery bypass graft (CABG) test (NCT00847964). Three months following Algisyl-LVR treatment has improved stroke volume and significantly reduced ESV and EDV among 3 and 6 months, The mean 6MWT test results were positive in the Algisyl-LVR implanted participants than untreated patients even after a year (NCT01311791). New York Heart Association (NYHA) sorting results at 6 and 12 months demonstrated 84–85% classification score in Algisyl-LVR treated group compared to the untreated group (25–26%) with a statistically non-significant benefit in LVM, LVEF, LVEDD and LVESD scores [10, 11]. Additionally clinical studies are undergoing testing the safety and efficiency of Algisyl-LVR in patients with serious heart failure (NCT03082508).

UMC Utrecht and Biosolution Co., Ltd. developed a cell-based treatment for patients with serious cartilage abnormalities [12]. A fibrin glue-based treatment mixed with combination of reprocessed autologous chondrons and allogenic MSCs (in 10:90 or 20:80 ratio) are given to patients in a Phase I clinical studies (NCT02037204). C-reactive protein can be seen at a lower level following seven days of treatment along with no FBR and reduced levels of erythrocyte sedimentation rate (ESR). Other important factors including Visual Analog Scale (VAS) average pain score was decreased following therapy. After 12 months of therapy, it was found that six out of ten patients have normal tissue restoration with another three closes to normal confirmed by arthroscopy and microscopic analysis. In their other studies with 35 participants were treated with similar technology for 18 months demonstrating a statistically significant decrease in the mean VAS pain score along with normal tissue restoration in 22 patients (NCT04236739) [13].

6.2 Conclusion and Future Perspectives

The sudden rise of various therapies directed towards tissue regeneration, immunotherapy, cell therapy, medical devices, tissue engineering, and organ implants, increase the necessity of biocompatible and immunocompatible delivery systems to control the host immune response, prevent FBR and improve the long-term therapeutic efficacy. Various methods were adopted to tune the surface characteristics of the biomaterials and chemical properties to obtained desired effects of long-term prevention of FBR and successful therapy associated with the tissue and cell engineering. It is significant to perceive that these methods are altered to the anticipated reaction and would vary according to their functions. This is an appealing choice allowing the utilization of immunomodulatory biomaterials for cell and tissue engineering applications including cell therapies in various diseases such as cancers, diabetes, cardiac diseases etc. Even though remarkable pre-clinical and clinical advancements are being made, more effort needs to do detailed toxicity, immunocompatibility, degradability studies testing these biomaterials rigorously before clinical approval. Even though some studies analyzed the influence of paracrine factors secreted from the cells in their overall toxicity and immune reactions, detailed analysis regarding fast or slow degrading materials in this context is missing. Systematic or rapid degradation of the biomaterial may change the therapeutic and immune responses and can have varying range of impacts on the outcome of the success or the failure of the therapy. A rapidly degrading biomaterials may be useful considering the fast delivery of the therapeutic drugs or molecules, whereas for long-term cell therapy one would aim to protect the cells with a non-degradable and immunoprotective biomaterials to facilitate the clinical outcomes. Chemical modifications of biomaterials need more research regarding leaching of chemical moieties that can have long term impacts on human body eliciting an immune or toxic responses. More studies are needed to develop customizable biomaterials that would be specific to certain applications that may not work well for others. Extensive collaboration among researchers from academia, industry and clinics are required to bridge the existing knowledge gap and facilitate this novel class of therapies to bring for the use of human curing several diseases.

References

1. Kim, B., Pradhan, L., Hernandez, A., Yenurkar, D., Nethi, S.K. and Mukherjee, S., Current Advances in Immunomodulatory Biomaterials for Cell Therapy and Tissue Engineering. *Advanced Therapeutics*, (2023), p. 2300002, https://doi.org/10.1002/adtp.202300002.
2. Mullard, A., 2023. FDA approves first cell therapy for type 1 diabetes. Nature Reviews Drug Discovery 22, 611 (2023) https://doi.org/10.1038/d41573-023-00113-w.
3. Vegas, A.J., Veiseh, O., Doloff, J.C., Ma, M., Tam, H.H., Bratlie, K., Li, J., Bader, A.R., Langan, E., Olejnik, K. and Fenton, P., Combinatorial hydrogel library enables identification of materials that mitigate the foreign body response in primates. *Nature biotechnology*, *34*(3), (2016), pp. 345-352.
4. Carlsson, P.O., Espes, D., Sedigh, A., Rotem, A., Zimerman, B., Grinberg, H., Goldman, T., Barkai, U., Avni, Y., Westermark, G.T. and Carlbom, L., Transplantation of macroencapsulated human islets within the bioartificial pancreas βAir to patients with type 1 diabetes mellitus. *American Journal of Transplantation*, *18*(7), (2018), pp. 1735-1744.
5. Debled, M., MacGrogan, G., Breton-Callu, C., Ferron, S., Hurtevent, G., Fournier, M., Bourdarias, L., Bonnefoi, H., Mauriac, L. and de Lara, C.T., Surgery following neoadjuvant chemotherapy for HER2-positive locally advanced breast cancer. Time to reconsider the standard attitude. *European Journal of Cancer*, *51*(6), (2015), pp. 697–704.
6. Menasché, P., Vanneaux, V., Hagège, A., Bel, A., Cholley, B., Parouchev, A., Cacciapuoti, I., Al-Daccak, R., Benhamouda, N., Blons, H. and Agbulut, O., Transplantation of human embryonic stem cell–derived cardiovascular progenitors for severe ischemic left ventricular dysfunction. *Journal of the American College of Cardiology*, *71*(4), (2018), pp. 429-438.
7. Frey, N., Linke, A., Süselbeck, T., Müller-Ehmsen, J., Vermeersch, P., Schoors, D., Rosenberg, M., Bea, F., Tuvia, S. and Leor, J., Intracoronary delivery of injectable bioabsorbable scaffold (IK-5001) to treat left ventricular remodeling after ST-elevation myocardial infarction: a first-in-man study. *Circulation: Cardiovascular Interventions*, *7*(6), (2014), pp. 806–812.
8. Rao, S.V., Zeymer, U., Douglas, P.S., Al-Khalidi, H., White, J.A., Liu, J., Levy, H., Guetta, V., Gibson, C.M., Tanguay, J.F. and Vermeersch, P., Bioabsorbable intracoronary matrix for prevention of ventricular remodeling after myocardial infarction. *Journal of the American College of Cardiology*, *68*(7), (2016), pp. 715-723.
9. Lee, L.C., Wall, S.T., Genet, M., Hinson, A. and Guccione, J.M., Bioinjection treatment: effects of post-injection residual stress on left ventricular wall stress. *Journal of Biomechanics*, *47*(12), (2014), pp. 3115-3119.

10. Ogle, B.M., Bursac, N., Domian, I., Huang, N.F., Menasché, P., Murry, C.E., Pruitt, B., Radisic, M., Wu, J.C., Wu, S.M. and Zhang, J., Distilling complexity to advance cardiac tissue engineering. *Science translational medicine*, 8(342), (2016), pp. 342ps13–342ps13.
11. McNally, E.M. and Mestroni, L., Dilated cardiomyopathy: genetic determinants and mechanisms. *Circulation research*, 121(7), (2017), pp. 731-748.
12. Monaco, G., El Haj, A.J., Alini, M. and Stoddart, M.J., Ex vivo systems to study chondrogenic differentiation and cartilage integration. *Journal of Functional Morphology and Kinesiology*, 6(1), (2021), p. 6.
13. de Windt, T.S., Vonk, L.A., Slaper-Cortenbach, I.C., Nizak, R., van Rijen, M.H. and Saris, D.B., Allogeneic MSCs and recycled autologous chondrons mixed in a one-stage cartilage cell transplantion: a first-in-man trial in 35 patients. *Stem cells*, 35(8), (2017), pp. 1984-1993.

The manufacturer's authorised representative in the EU is Springer Nature Customer Service Centre GmbH, Europaplatz 3, 69115 Heidelberg, Germany. If you have any concerns regarding our products, please contact ProductSafety@springernature.com

Printed and bound by CPI Group (UK) Ltd, Croydon, CR0 4YY

26/03/2026

02078953-0019